Row, Row, Row

My Boat!

A WOMAN'S INCREDIBLE JOURNEY

WITH

BREAST CANCER

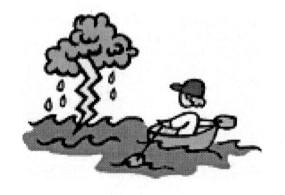

Margreet Jansen van Doorn

Trafford Publishing/ Victoria

Author's Note
This book was written about my personal experience
with breast cancer and to let you know that being
actively involved in your own healing journey is a
gift you can give yourself. It is NOT designed to take
you away from whatever healing or health program you
are on – whether it is mainstream or alternative. In the
field of healing there are no guarantees, and there
are as many ways to healing and health as there are
people. Hopefully, my story will inspire and support
you in whatever path you choose.

Note for Librarians: A cataloguing record for this book is available from Library and Archives
Canada at www.collectionscanada.ca/amicus/index-e.html
ISBN 1-4120-7993-4

*Printed in Victoria, BC, Canada. Printed on paper with minimum 30% recycled fibre. Trafford's print shop
runs on "green energy" from solar, wind and other environmentally-friendly power sources.*

TRAFFORD
PUBLISHING™
Offices in Canada, USA, Ireland and UK
This book was published *on-demand* in cooperation with Trafford Publishing. On-demand
publishing is a unique process and service of making a book available for retail sale to the
public taking advantage of on-demand manufacturing and Internet marketing. On-demand
publishing includes promotions, retail sales, manufacturing, order fulfilment, accounting and
collecting royalties on behalf of the author.

Book sales for North America and international:
Trafford Publishing, 6E–2333 Government St.,
Victoria, BC V8T 4P4 CANADA
phone 250 383 6864 (toll-free 1 888 232 4444)
fax 250 383 6804; email to orders@trafford.com
Book sales in Europe:
Trafford Publishing (UK) Limited, 9 Park End Street, 2nd Floor
Oxford, UK OX1 1HH UNITED KINGDOM
phone 44 (0)1865 722 113 (local rate 0845 230 9601)
facsimile 44 (0)1865 722 868; info.uk@trafford.com
Order online at:
trafford.com/05-2891

10 9 8 7 6 5 4

This Book is dedicated in loving memory to my parents:
Tony and Steven,

my mother, Anthonia Margaretha Jansen van Doorn,
for teaching me that all you have to do is ask and you can get "yes";

my father, Steven Nardus Jansen van Doorn,
for showing me the adventures you find by taking roads less traveled.

Life is a gift.
Live Now!

Margreet

Contents

Prologue

L ife and death are intricately interwoven. They belong together; one does not exist exclusively without the other. For every life there is a death. In life, death walks beside us every day, except we mostly do not think about it. It is often only when we are faced with a serious illness that we are reminded. It is almost as if death taps us on the shoulder and says, "Here is a reminder: I am right beside you!"

Most of us then become frightened because we seem to suddenly become aware that death is there, walking right next to us, not realizing that death was there all along....

It is much the same how the stars and moon are present during the day. Usually we don't realize they're there because in the day's brightness they are not visible. We say the stars and moon only come "out" at night because we only see them in the dark; yet, they are always "out" not just at night, but also during the day.

So it is for death. It is also always there, but we usually do not acknowledge it, until our world turns dark, when we have been diagnosed with a potentially fatal illness, that death is right beside us!

Chapter One

Finding a lump

BEING ALONE

This part of my story began one Sunday evening. It was after 11:30pm on April 30, 1996, and I was standing in front of the bathroom mirror looking at my reflection and feeling unhappy with my life and what I looked like. I had gained far too much weight, had not had a haircut in a long time, and I felt very unattractive. To compound my misery, I was thinking that I had been alone for such a long time and felt that my fate was to be alone, forever: I was feeling very lonely. My 38th birthday had just passed and middle age was looming. Money was tight. I had recently bought my first house, a third of a nice triplex, and I had also bought my first new car months earlier, but the pressures of both a car loan and a mortgage were wearing me down. The continual struggle from having been a single mom for almost a decade and a half was beginning to take its toll. Life seemed very bleak. I had a case of PLOM disease—Poor Little Old Me!

Shortly before midnight on a Sunday evening, there was not much I could do about most of that; however, there was one thing I could change that evening—my hair! I looked down on the counter and saw that beside me lay a pair of scissors. I decided to give myself a trim. I must have been a little more zealous in my cutting than I thought because after I had cut my hair, I noticed that it looked quite a bit shorter than I had been wearing it, but I liked it. I also saw that there was a narrow strand hanging down the back of my neck. It was noticeably longer than the rest and it needed to be cut, yet as hard as I tried, I could not reach it.

I had made more noise than I thought because I had not meant to wake him up, but it was then that my son Vincent came out of his room. He looked very sleepy. He mumbled, "Mom, what are you doing?" I told him that I had been cutting my hair, and I explained to him about the strand I could not reach, and then I handed him the scissors.

What possessed me to give those scissors to my 14-year-old, sleepy, teenage son could only be called temporary insanity. But I did give the scissors to him with the instructions to cut the very thin strand of longer hair at the nape of my neck. It should have been very easy for him and should not have taken him very long....

Well, he began to cut. He moved slowly because he was barely awake. I was obviously not too swift myself; however, that changed rapidly when I heard him mutter," Mom you have so much hair." I was just about to reply and ask him what he meant by that when he handed me an amount of hair which filled the palm of his hand. It was much more than a very thin long strand. I looked at it horrified and yelled, near tears, "What have you done?"

He had cut my hair, but not the thin strand I had imagined he would. He had, half asleep, cut a handful of hair from the back of my head. I tried to find a mirror so I could look at the "damage," but could not find any: Although it was not visible to me yet, he had carefully cut a large U shape into my hair into the nape of my neck. I now had a very unique hairstyle certainly not yet discovered by the Fashion Police. The gloom I had been feeling earlier was nothing compared to the wretchedness that washed over me.

I thought, "I'm fat, middle aged, broke, alone, tired, and now I have a strange haircut." I felt totally miserable! I experienced a hopeless feeling of grinding despair with the state of my life. Feeling this way, I could not think of anything positive about my life. It was now very late, well past midnight, and I had to get up early later that day to go to my job. It was time to go to bed; I would just try to sleep; maybe after a good night's rest, everything would not seem so bad in the morning. That was something my mother had always told me, and it was something I had already passed on to Vincent, "Everything always seems worse at night!"

I brushed my teeth, put my nightgown on, and went to bed. I tried to find a comfortable place to sleep, still feeling very sorry for myself and with my miserable life. I tossed and turned and turned and tossed until finally I ended up lying on my left side. It was after I stopped moving, when I was trying to relax and get calm, that it felt as if I had rolled on something hard. It felt like a piece of stone, but since my mattress was old and lumpy I assumed that I had landed on a lumpy part of the mattress. I shifted to another part of the bed but felt "the piece of stone" again. It seemed as if the stone had moved with me, or had it? Everything that happened next appeared to move in slow motion; time seemed somehow suspended. It was as if someone took my hand and placed it under my left breast. My fingers almost automatically went to the spot where I had rolled on the "stone." And then, time came crashing back, reality hit me square in the face, my breath caught in my throat: My hand had found a lump!

Immediately I was wide-awake! I turned on the light and touched the area on the underside of my breast with my other hand. It was as if I was hoping that my one hand had been "wrong" and my other hand would be "right" and not feel anything. But no such luck: I felt it again; there was definitely something solid under my skin! It felt hard, and it felt large—about the size of a dove egg (1" x ¾" or 2 ½ x 1 ½ cm). I waited a few minutes trying not to panic, trying to take a deep breath, willing myself to be calm. Then, tentatively, I touched IT again, still hoping that a few minutes earlier I had been wrong, that I had only imagined finding something. But IT was still there!

I tried hard not to panic, but my thoughts immediately went to the big "C" word: I felt certain that was what I had found.

13

Forgotten were my sorry feelings for myself, my money worries, being a single parent, my problems with overeating, my hair. I was convinced in those early midnight hours that I had found a cancerous lump in my left breast. Alone in those dark hours of the night, with no one to tell me differently, I saw myself losing my newly purchased house and my new car; yet, somehow that didn't seem to matter too much. I was now face to face with a deadly foe and there was a strong chance that my life could be over, that I could die! And I realized that I did not want to die. As much as I had disliked my life earlier, I did want life, not anyone else's life. I acknowledged that I wanted my own life, complete with all its challenges. I did not want it to end.

Like a thief in the night, so I would not wake Vincent again, I tip toed downstairs to my bookcase to try and find my Medical Book so I could read what it said under breast lumps. I looked all over the bookcase, but I could not find the book there, so I went back upstairs again, where, after quietly yet frantically searching my bedroom, I finally found the book under my bed. I quickly found the chapter I needed. I read that most breast lumps are cysts, but the book also explained that a breast lump could be cancer. I desperately tried to stay calm by repeatedly telling myself, "Wait until the morning; make a doctor's appointment. Don't panic; go to sleep. Everything will look better in the morning." But I wasn't sure if it would be. I was very afraid.

I did not sleep much that night. It took a long time before I finally fell asleep just before dawn, and the sleep I managed to 'steal' was anything but rejuvenating. Waking up was not a slow process that morning. I was instantly awake, and my first thought was about the frightening discovery I had made. I knew I had to check it. Perhaps I had been asleep and had imagined everything. And so again I moved my hand slowly toward my breast, hoping that it had all been a dream and 'IT' would not be there. But once more my fingers felt the thickening under my skin: IT was still there…! This was not a dream; finding a lump was not something I had imagined; life, for me, had indeed changed the night before.

For a minute I felt paralyzed: What should I do? But then I came up with a plan, an action I could take.

I would go and see my doctor; maybe she could reassure me. Maybe she would not even find anything; maybe she would not be able to feel the lump my fingers were touching. Maybe there was still the possibility that it was all my imagination.

Soon, Vincent woke up. I did not tell him of my frightening discovery. I didn't want to worry him 'needlessly. "I got dressed and waited until Vincent was safely off to school before I phoned the health clinic to see if I could come in and see my doctor. The receptionist who picked up the phone answered that my doctor was very busy and the earliest appointment available to me would be in three days, on Thursday. But today was only Monday. The receptionist did not ask me why I needed an appointment. So, perhaps for no other reason than to hear myself say it, I told her matter of factly that I had found a lump in my breast. It got her attention instantly and this seemed to change everything. She told me to come in immediately, no appointment was necessary; she would fit me in as soon as I got there!

Frightened even more by the receptionist's obvious concern, I now found myself stalling. A part of me wanted to race to the health clinic to the place where I could find answers, but there was yet another part who really did not want to know. Ignorance is bliss! As long as I did not involve another person, I could pretend that it was all my imagination. Right now, it only existed in my mind. And so I stalled. I cleaned up the kitchen first, washed the dishes, put them away, then dusted off my computer; next, I rearranged the shoes by the front door: All things I normally would not do. They were insignificant things I felt compelled to do before I finally drove to the health clinic.

I walked slowly inside the building and even slower toward the receptionist. I told her my name and why I was there and that I did not have an appointment. Her face immediately showed great concern and she asked me if I had called earlier that morning; I told her I had. Again her reaction filled me with anxiety. She seemed to take this so seriously. I wanted her to look at me without seeing me and tell me with that bland, slightly bored look she had always given me in the past that I should go and wait in the waiting room until the doctor could see me. Today, she did not look at me that way: She looked worried. Her face mirrored what I was feeling. She seemed human this time when she told me compassionately to wait in the waiting room.

I forced myself to walk calmly to the waiting room. While there, thoughts raced through my head, "why am I here?", "I'm probably imagining all of this and I should just leave.", "My Doctor won't find anything anyway, and I'm probably overreacting." Sitting there, in the waiting room, on a Monday morning with a painless lump in my breast seemed surreal. I was thinking to myself that I should be at work, not here in this place, wasting time at a doctor's office. I had waited approximately 15 minutes continuously debating with myself, and I finally convinced myself to leave. I was getting ready to get up and walk out of the waiting room, when my name was called. I was taken to an examining room where the nurse asked me why I was there. When I told her, she, too, seemed instantly concerned. More gentle than usual, she told me to undress from the waist up and to put on a paper gown.

I didn't have to wait long because I had just finished putting on the gown when my doctor walked into the small room. We greeted each other and talked for a few minutes about superficial matters. Seeing her face reassured me somewhat. This doctor, my doctor, would make it all OK. I had felt truly blessed when I had found her, seven years earlier in a small office in a strip mall. She was the kind of doctor who was not afraid to show her humanity. Her bedside manner was caring and sensitive. She had recently moved to the large medical centre we were now at, but it was her mannerism and caring nature that had made me follow her and put up with the barriers the receptionist and nurses placed around her. Seeing her usually made me forget that I had been placed on hold for over 10 minutes before I could request an appointment, and that it was often nearly impossible to see her the same day, or that once I had an appointment I had to wait at least another 15 – 20 minutes before I was taken to an examination room. She was here now and would certainly tell me everything was OK.

She asked me to lay down on the table, and when I had done so she did a breast examination. I waited for her to tell me that it was nothing and give me a simple medical term and send me home. But that was not what happened: the examination seemed to take longer, and when she finished she looked up at me. In my hypersensitive state, I noticed that she hesitated slightly before she spoke. Then she told me that she too could feel something in my left breast. Reality: I was not asleep, I was not imagining the lump, my imagination had not created this, and this was real! I now had proof because my doctor could feel it too. I swallowed hard.

My doctor, the wonderful, warm, caring, compassionate professional she is, immediately noticed my anxiety and tried to be comforting. She explained that, a month earlier, during my annual physical, she had performed a breast exam and had not found anything, so most likely this was probably a cyst. She clarified that cysts can appear seemingly overnight, and since this was a fairly large lump, which she had not felt a month earlier, she was quite certain this was a cyst. She then asked me if my period was about to start, and I told her it was. "All signs that it probably is a cyst," she replied. She also let me know that she herself had just had a lump removed earlier in the year and hers had been a cyst. But she continued by informing me that, as a precaution, I should go for a mammogram, anyway. She said, "Just to cover all the bases."

She gave me a requisition form for a mammogram with instructions that it was better to wait and go after my period had started and was almost over. She did not tell me why and I did not ask. By not asking the rationale behind this, I eagerly accepted the welcome postponement of having to face more reality.

I left my doctor's office, not at all comforted by her assurance that this was probably a cyst. Something inside me continued faintly whispering the "C" word. It was not a loud sound; it was more like a faint, troublesome murmur. I had not yet become used to listening to this small voice inside me, so for the most part I ignored it. But it kept whispering, nagging, murmuring, and constantly stirring in my thoughts. I decided not to tell anyone about my frightening discovery. I had always handled whatever came my way, alone. I would handle this too, by myself. Besides, I reasoned, who could I tell?

Marian, my oldest sister, who had been my friend longer than anyone else, had enough on her plate. Her daughter had been diagnosed with, and was still being treated for, leukemia. My other sister and close friend, Anneke, with whom I share a very special bond, was in the final stages of her second pregnancy. I couldn't worry her, especially since she had been through a cancer scare with her husband in 1989. That left my remaining siblings and Pa; I was not particularly close to any of them at that time. My closest bond had been with my mother. But I couldn't tell her: she had died 7 years earlier. I had two other sisters, both younger than me. There was Joan, my youngest sister, whose mother-in-law had just died of cancer, and who had, months earlier, delivered twin girls. And there was Liesbeth my other sister. I was not close enough to either of them at that time to turn to them for comfort or guidance.

And so by mentally calling to mind each of my siblings, I reasoned that I could not tell any of my sisters—the timing was just not right. That left my dad and my brother. Talking about having found a lump in my breast? No, that was not something I would talk to my younger brother about: in my mind, he was still my baby brother, even though he had turned 30 that year. And then there was my dad. At this point I had totally convinced myself they would all worry needlessly, so I kept the information to myself. I put the form with the mammogram request in my purse, where it would stay for a week, ticking like a time bomb. I also did not tell any friends; I spoke to no one about what I was facing—but it was never out of my thoughts.

The rest of that Monday, I joked with everyone about my hair, using the diversion technique. If I talked and laughed about my "strange hair," then I didn't have to talk about having a lump growing in my breast. I didn't want to talk about it, and I kept trying not to think about it. But the fact remained that a lump had grown in my left breast, and it continued growing. It had not been there at all a month before, and now it seemed to have a life of its own.

I could stop myself from talking about it, but I could not stop myself from thinking about IT! Many times I would be in the middle of a conversation with colleagues, or friends, when a part of me wanted to blurt out, "Guess what, I found a lump in my breast." With morbid, detached curiosity a part of me wanted to see what people's reaction would be. Would it stop the conversation? Would they gasp with fear? Would they, too, tell me it was probably a cyst? I'll never know, because I didn't speak of it to anyone during that long week. And so there it stayed as a closely guarded secret.

It was Saturday, when I finally began to speak my thoughts. Voltaire said, "We employ speech to conceal our thoughts." Well, I had effectively done just that for six days. It was in the morning when my close friend Jenni called. We talked for a few minutes about other things and then I told her, trying to sound very matter of factly, what I had found the Sunday before. Jenni was already an important person in my support system, and not yet known to me, she would soon become even more important. Her reaction was somewhat soothing: she did not appear overly concerned and she told me that these things were mostly cysts and that she had had one removed when she was in her early twenties. I did feel somewhat comforted by her words, but did not feel reassured. However, I realized that it helped me to talk to a caring person about my worry, even if it made the lump seem more real.

Next, I told Vincent, and this time I reassured him that it was nothing to worry about and that our doctor thought it was a cyst. It was, of course, a false reassurance—something I did not feel at all myself. A part of me, deep down, did know that this was not a cyst, that IT was the big "C."

Later that day, Pa came for a visit. We usually play a few games of cards when my dad visits, and during a cribbage card game, I started to tell him several times of my frightening discovery, but each time I let myself be interrupted by a side conversation. After I had told Vincent about the lump growing in my breast he had asked if anyone else knew. I had told him no. Then he had said that I should tell Pa. He reasoned, and of course was right, "He is your dad and he should know." Kids are often very wise. . . . We had a nice visit, the three of us, and then it was time for Pa to leave. I had still not said anything about finding a lump in my breast. I walked him to his car, and I tried to speak, trying to tell him very matter of factly. But this time my pseudo calm façade began to crack, and I knew I was very close to crying. After all, this was my Pa. But I decided that tears would make it seem far worse, so I choked them back, and soon was in control again. I still had not told him. I wanted to formulate the "proper" words, so the information would be buffered, but I could not think of how to do that. I was afraid that if I waited again, I would not be able to tell him. There was no way around it: I just had to do it.

"Pa, I found a lump." I blurted out.

He did not respond immediately, as if to fully comprehend what I had just said. I could see shock begin to register on his face. "In your breast?" he asked tentatively. I nodded, both of us knowing that we remembered my mom's younger sister who, at 36, had died from breast cancer. I was barely two years older, at 38. I tried to shield him from the fear and the memory, or perhaps it was me that I tried to shield, instead. I did not want him to think about her; I did not want to think about her, so I tried to cover her memory by telling my dad that my doctor thought it was probably a cyst. Pa nodded in agreement, all too eager to believe what a doctor had said, but the fear stayed in his eyes.

"Have you told your sisters?"

"No. "

"Is it OK if I let them know?"

"Yeah. "

We stood there by his car for a few moments, not knowing what else to say. Then I kissed Pa on his weathered cheek;

although I'm tall, I had to stand on my toes to do this because he is a very big man. He kissed me back and got into his car. We looked at each other and I could see that the fear was still in his eyes. Mutely, we waved to each other as he drove away.

And that night, one after the other, all my siblings phoned me, and I, who had always felt that I should carry all my burdens alone, felt comforted and nurtured and part of the large family I belong to. Perhaps allowing others to help was OK, after all?

Chapter Two

Getting a mammogram

ISOLATION DEEPENS. BETRAYAL. INDIFFERENCE

The next day, another Sunday, my period started, so on Monday I phoned the clinic where I was to have my mammogram. I was told that they had an opening that week. This seemed far too soon. I wanted to go, but I was not sure I was "ready" to go that week. I was just becoming accustomed to the idea that I had a lump. I wanted to process it a bit longer. Strangely, I wanted to delay discovering what it was by postponing having a mammogram. Of course, I realized that this was not logical at all because I knew it was important that the lump was checked. But logic does not always rule in times of crises and fear.

Not wanting to say any of this to the person answering the phone, I asked for the next available appointment after that. I was told that there wasn't another opening for at least another two weeks. So even though I felt conflicted, I decided to let logic prevail by accepting the appointment for that week. Sometimes circumstance saves us from ourselves.

By now, I had begun to tell people, colleagues and friends, about the lump I had found in my breast. After talking with people, it seemed that everyone knew someone who had a lump, and all those lumps had been cysts. Marian, my sister, told me that she too had found a lump, only a few months earlier. Her lump had been tested, and she found out, when a needle had been inserted and fluid was extracted, that her lump had been a cyst. But even with everyone telling me their stories of cysts and trying to reassure me, the feeling inside me continued to grow stronger with the certainty that my lump was not a cyst!

The day of my mammogram appointment arrived; I went to the clinic inside the mall and sat in the waiting room in a daze, thinking, "This day could change my life." I looked around me, detachedly, at the other women waiting there. Were they here for the same reason I was? Had they, too, found a lump, or were they here for routine mammograms? I had never had a mammogram before because I was too young to be in the age group where they recommend that you have them. I had only just turned 38 years old in March. Most doctors recommend you have your first mammogram at 50. Some feel it is a good idea to have a base line done at 40. I was still two years short of any need for a mammogram.

Because I had never had a mammogram before, I didn't know what to expect. I had heard that mammograms were painful, and I felt anxious, but I also continued to feel removed from everything. This was not happening to me, surely it wasn't? Was I in shock?

After some time passed, I was called in and told to change into a paper gown to get ready for my mammogram. I was taken into a small room where the machine loomed. The technician asked me to stand up against it. The machine felt very cold against my skin. My breast was put between what looked like two ironing boards. A knob was turned and the ironing boards were squeezed very tight. It hurt a lot! It was now very difficult for me to stay detached; the pain had catapulted me right back into the present, into the room where one after the other my breasts were being squeezed until they hurt so much I wanted to scream. I could feel the tears begin to form, but I closed my eyes and so held them in check. I was going to be strong.

It seemed like an eternity before this ordeal was over. What had felt like torture was finally finished. The technician told me to wait until the doctor present had been able to view the x-ray. She told me not to get dressed, yet until everything was clear and she would give me the signal. I was told to return to and wait in the little cubbyhole. In a little paper gown with just enough space for me to sit, I mutely stared at the door. I needed human comfort, a human voice telling me it was going to be OK, a shoulder to lean on, a hand on my back, anything. Instead, nothing: I was alone behind a closed door, shivering in that thin throw-away paper gown.

After 10 minutes, the technician came back and said I had to come back into another room. The doctor also wanted me to have an ultrasound. She told me not to worry—they just wanted to be sure. But I was worried and I had so many questions tumble around in my mind. What was this ultrasound about? And who were "they"? No one offered me information and I did not want to ask. I did not want to be a nuisance. I was strong, I could face this quickly, alone, and then I would rush home and process everything there or try to push it away, pretend it was not happening to me. I would do this in my usual way—I would read a book, or watch TV, knit, use anything to distract my mind. Incidentally, I had just started reading a book about the Ebola virus. In my mind I reasoned that compared to what happened to people who had contracted the Ebola virus, what I was possibly facing paled in comparison. I tried to convince myself that, after all it could always be worse....

Having the ultrasound done did not hurt at all, and after it was taken, I was again told to return to the little change cubby hole. Again, I was told not to get dressed. I continued feeling very alone. The waiting felt like another eternity. Minutes moved like snails. Thirty long minutes passed before someone came to get me again. Once more, I had to come back in because they wanted to take another mammogram. This one was to focus exclusively on the lump, enlarging it. Again I was told by the technician not to worry. She said that, based on her experience, what was sitting in my breast looked like a cyst. Everyone involved was now in agreement that they could see a mass with a clearly defined outline. The woman explained that it did not have the ragged undefined edges which are characteristic of cancer.

Again, I had to stand up against the cold machine, and this

time only my left breast, was squeezed between the "ironing boards." By now, however, I knew what to expect and it was a little less physically traumatic. As for my emotional state, that was quite a different matter. I was feeling very anxious. After the picture, I had to wait again for a sign of dismissal before getting dressed. This time it was finally offered and I was allowed to leave. The technician's parting comment to me as I was leaving was for me not to worry. I thought, "Is she trying to covertly tell me something?" "Is she making an effort to give me hope?" It was a hope I did not feel! My inner knowing continued to grow stronger. I began to realize with more certainty that I already knew, and had known from the moment when I first felt it, what this lump really was. And it was not a cyst....

A few agonizing days passed, full of worry about what the tests would reveal. Needing to do something, anything, I finally phoned my doctor's office to see if the results were back. I spoke to my doctor's nurse and she explained that they had not come in yet, but she promised to call me as soon as they arrived. So all I could do was wait; this kind of waiting to find out about the results of my mammogram was sheer agony. I wasn't sure what I would be told, but speculating and not knowing anything with certainty was even more difficult. So many variables were possible, and in my mind I was going over all of them continuously. And so a few more difficult days passed, filled with guessing. Finally, after I felt that I would never find out the answer, my doctor's office called. I was asked if I could come in as soon as possible because the results of my mammogram had come back. All in all, more than a week had passed. It had been an incredibly trying week. I had not been able to sleep well, and I felt like I had aged hundreds of years from worry.

I made an appointment, again: more waiting in the waiting room before I was taken in a room and until my doctor entered. But I felt certain I would be given some useful information, so I continued waiting patiently. But when she finally came in and gave me the results, her news was frustrating. All she was able to tell me was that now it was confirmed that there was something in my breast. We now had proof because it was showing up on the mammogram. I was stunned; I felt like saying, "Well, we knew that; we could feel it with our fingers, couldn't we?" Did I have to wait a week to have confirmed what both of us had already been able to touch? But I didn't say anything because I had always been taught to respect and listen to my doctor and not to question what she told me.

The next step, she told me, would be to see, whether what everyone (including my doctor) thought was a cyst could be drained. My doctor's nurse would call me with an appointment the next day. The next day would be Thursday. By now, almost two drawn-out weeks had passed since I had first felt the lump. Again I had to deal with more waiting, more time to speculate, more time for uncertainty. I tried very hard not to worry during that next waiting period, but it was very difficult.

I tried to think about and concentrate on other things. It was not easy. However, a welcome distraction was arriving shortly. My friend Ieke, from Holland, was coming for a visit soon and she would stay at my house. It was something I had eagerly anticipated. We had not seen each other for seven years. Nonetheless, my excitement about her pending visit was now seriously overshadowed by my current fears.

The next day Thursday, I decided to work from home so I could stay close to the phone and not miss the promised call from my doctor's nurse. It was very hard to concentrate on work; I know I did not get much done. I waited all day, but no phone call came! Another day had been spent worrying, speculating, thinking the unthinkable.

Friday, I decided to take matters into my own hands and at the end of the morning, around noon, I called my doctor's office. I was put on hold for more than 10 minutes by the main reception and when the receptionist finally came back on the line she told me that my doctor and her nurse had left for the day. She ended the call by asking me, without listening for the answer, if I could phone back on Monday.

I felt stunned! Why had my doctor's nurse not called me the day before, Thursday, as promised? Why had she not taken a few seconds to phone me, even if it was only to tell me she had not been able to get me an appointment yet? It appeared obvious that she had made the promise without considering what all this waiting was doing to me. I was now so frustrated I wanted to scream, but the person I wanted to yell at had left for the day. She had gone home without any thought that I was waiting in fear for her call.

Yet, there was nothing I could do but wait some more. The weekend was now looming ahead. It turned out to be one of the longest weekends of my life. Seconds moved like hours, minutes felt like infinity, which made the days almost impossible to get through. I was still trying not to worry, but couldn't help it. Again, I tried to fill my time with diversions, but no diversion was strong enough to distract me.

I, who had always been very good at ignoring how I felt and pushing away uncomfortable feelings and fears, was now no longer able to do so.

After what had seemed like another eternity, the weekend was finally over. I woke up early on Monday morning and promptly at 9 o'clock, the moment the Medical Center opened, I phoned my doctor's office. As usual, I was put on hold—not surprisingly, for more than 10 minutes. When the receptionist finally returned and after I asked to be connected to my doctor's nurse, I was told that my doctor and her nurse were not in that day. Once more, I felt numb and stunned and so incredibly betrayed. I wanted to yell and scream and throw a full-blown temper tantrum. I wanted to ask the uncheerful, unapproachable, unfriendly receptionist, "Why did the person answering the phone on Friday not tell me then that my doctor and her nurse would also not be in on Monday?" I had barely survived the weekend.

The only way I had made it through Saturday and Sunday was the thought that it would soon be Monday and then I would be able to talk to someone in my doctor's office. I didn't know who to be angriest at, which didn't make a difference, anyway, because no one seemed to be available for me to vent my frustration. I felt thoroughly disillusioned by my doctor's nurse's actions or lack of courtesy, the uncooperative receptionist, even my own doctor—surely she had to know what her staff was doing to her patients? My trust in the entire Medical Community was shaken. My confidence in them was being tested. I made a decision at that moment—I decided not to call my doctor's office anymore. This was too hard! Every time I had tried calling my doctor, I had needed more and more nerve to do so and had become more and more upset. I would no longer do that to myself; I would not put myself through more agony. Yet, I still had no answer and the worry over my health continued.

The next day, Tuesday, five very long days after the promised date, my doctor's nurse finally phoned me to give me the appointment date and time. I did not tell her about the long days and nights I had spent agonizing, worrying, waiting for her call and the frustration I felt with her and everyone connected with the Medical Clinic where my doctor has her office. She did not apologize or even seem to realize what I had been through as a result of her broken promise and that, originally, she had told me that she would phone me the previous Thursday.

For now, this part of the waiting, the waiting to get an appointment date, was over, and I did feel some relief. At least something was moving; I now, finally, had a date.

I recognized the date. May 21. It was a date I had looked forward to for awhile. It was the same day that my friend Ieke would arrive from Holland. Not only was my appointment on the same day, but it was also in the afternoon around the same time Ieke arrived. It would not give me enough time to meet her at the airport. I was told that my appointment was for the next Tuesday at 2:40pm. Ieke's plane was scheduled to arrive that same day at 2:30pm. I would have to make alternative arrangements to have Ieke picked up.

As fate would have it, that night, one of Ieke's friends called me. She wanted to know whether I was going to the airport to pick Ieke up or whether she should. I asked if she could go and gave the reason why. "Oh," she said, "I get cysts all the time." Like everyone else, she, too, was positive that my lump would be a cyst. By now I was just letting people talk about their cysts; it was as if they were trying to convince themselves—it no longer felt as if it had anything to do with me. I realized that they were addressing their own fears.

Meanwhile, Pa asked if I wanted him to go with me to my appointment, but I had not yet allowed myself to be helped by others so I told him that I didn't think it was necessary. Once more I would go alone, my choice—I still behaved like Jane Wayne. I felt that I could handle what life sent me, alone. I would discover, later, that it was so much better to have another person beside you, even if it is to sit in silence together. But at that time, I was still resisting offers of help from people.

Chapter Three

More testing

MORE DISTANCE

Now that I finally had a date for my appointment, it seemed that time was rushing again, and it felt like the day of my appointment arrived too soon. That Tuesday, May 21, I did some work in the morning, and then I went home for lunch. I was feeling very restless, and it was difficult to eat, so I decided that since I had to wait I would go to my appointment early and just wait there. I would sit in the waiting room and just read some of the gossip magazines. I arrived at the mall parking lot at twenty after two. It was twenty minutes before my appointment time. I walked into the clinic at twenty-five after two, still fifteen minutes ahead of my allotted time of 2:40. I explained to the receptionist that I was early. I'm never early for anything and I consider myself an "On Timer," which means that when I have an appointment or a meeting, I arrive on the agreed upon time—not early, not late, but right on time! This is why I felt I had to announce to the receptionist that I was early.

An angry looking woman in a white lab coat who was standing next to the receptionist and who had been looking down into the appointment book, looked up and contradicted me, "NO!," she said, sounding quite irritated, "YOU ARE LATE! YOUR APPOINTMENT WAS AT 2:15!" My heart sank. Her tone and her manner made me feel like a schoolgirl who was being scolded. I felt small and vulnerable, and severely chastised for being "late." But how could that be? I wasn't late, I was early. I knew that I could not have made a mistake. I would not have written down the wrong information for such an important appointment: 2:15 did not even sound like 2:40. If the time my doctor's nurse had given me had been 2:50 it could have been possible that I had misunderstood and had mixed up 2:15 with 2:50. But mistaking 2:15 for 2:40 did not make any sense. I kept going over it in my mind but could not understand it. The only thing that made any sense at all was that I had been given the wrong time by my doctor's nurse.

How this was possible I don't know. Had she been given the wrong time, or had she been so busy that she had given me the wrong time? That I will never know. It was most unfortunate for me, because I was at the receiving end of the technician's irritation with my perceived lateness and this did nothing to decrease my own already raised anxiety level; in fact, it elevated it even more. I was now utterly rattled.

I tried to explain to her, apologetically, that I had been given the wrong time. She seemed to sneer at this. Her attitude seemed to convey that nurses do not give patients wrong times, ever! The problem had to have been mine. She did not even appear to listen to what I was saying, and just looked at me as if I were trying to make up excuses for being late. This is how I interpreted the look of "yeah right" on her face. She appeared to be indulging in the fact that yet another patient was making her wait, not even attempting to give any thought to what I could possibly be feeling. Her only concern seemed to be that I had inconvenienced her.

At this point, the emotional strain had accumulated to an unbearable weight. I, who could usually contain my tears, could feel them dangerously close to the surface. But I was not going to cry in front of this irritated woman. I swallowed hard and tried to concentrate on my breathing—anything so I would not burst into tears. It worked only a little.

I was immediately taken to a little cubbyhole change room identical to the one where I had spent so much time the day of my mammogram. I was once again given a thin, short, paper gown and told to change into it.

A voice in my head was beginning to hiss at me. It was a voice of anxiety, not the voice of my heart I would later listen to. It nagged, it questioned, it prodded with the following, "Was there a message in the mix up of my appointment time?" I tried not to think that this could be a "sign" and it that it meant that I was not just late for my appointment but that I was also 'late' for my health. Would I be getting a death sentence soon? The thought continued to nag, like a cartoon devil sitting on my shoulder, maliciously hissing in my ear. But it wasn't a devil; these were my own ideas—they were not originating outside of me, they came from inside. I tried to ignore them, but they stubbornly kept returning. So many thoughts were racing through my head, so many feelings were competing for dominance, fear, uneasiness, discomfort, worry, anxiety, and frustration. I tried to stop my thinking altogether, but this was an impossibility. I changed fast into the gown, to make things easier for the medical people I had so severely inconvenienced by my perceived "lateness."

I was taken into a dimly lit room, where I was told to lay on a cot. I was told to take off my paper gown and was given a paper sheet. Then I braced myself for more waiting. Covered with only a thin sheet of paper, I was naked from the waist up. It felt like I was in that room, alone, for a long time—it was probably not more than ten minutes. Yet, the wait felt more like ten hours. I felt exposed, cold, and vulnerable. A paper sheet does very little to cover you or keep you warm.

Finally, a doctor and an assistant came into the room—two women. The female doctor explained the procedure and then immediately proceeded to do it. She assumed I had no questions. At this point, I was feeling quite numb, cold, and very afraid. Neither she, nor her assistant, appeared to be aware of me, the person, or of the fact that I was a living, breathing human being. I could have been a corpse.

After giving me a light, local freezing, the doctor inserted a needle into the lump with an attempt to drain it. I could not see what they were doing—it did not feel very uncomfortable, but I was still cold. I was trying to concentrate on getting warm when I heard the doctor say the following words—I'm not sure to whom she was speaking, because it certainly did not feel directed at me; her words cut through me like a knife; they made me forget how cold and uncomfortable I was, "It is not a cyst!"

And my world shattered!

The reassuring words I had heard so often during the last few weeks were now splashed all over the room! Everyone had tried to comfort me, to reassure, to give me hope that my lump was probably a cyst, and now this woman and her assistant had ripped hope away from me by uttering these five little words: "IT IS NOT A CYST!"

Simultaneously, the words stamped themselves into my mind, and I felt tears flood my eyes. I had to swallow hard, telling myself that I was not going to cry in this cold room, in front of these unfriendly, seemingly unfeeling people. I felt like I was part of a lab experiment. Besides, they had not given me any form of human comfort so far, so I certainly did not expect any empathy from them now, if I were to cry.

I did not feel safe to show my vulnerability. I still felt that to them I was just a body with a lump, not a living person with feelings and a personality. They did not know me, nor did they appear to want to find out who I was, let alone how I was doing. I had inconvenienced them. I stared hard at the ceiling, trying to find a spot I could focus on so I would not begin to sob. I was biting my lip, hard, then my tongue, trying to will myself to push back the ever-growing flood of tears in my eyes. But I couldn't do it; the tears kept coming. I wanted to close my eyes so I could absorb the tears. All my concentration went to not wanting to cry in front of these two women, and hearing inside my head repeated over and over again the words, "It is NOT a cyst!"

As if the doctor had read my thoughts, she now spoke more compassionately than before. She even looked toward my face, but not quite right at me when she said, "That doesn't mean anything, yet; there is a whole range of what it could be before it is cancer," and she proceeded to name them, all of which I have long forgotten because I was not really listening to that part of what she said. A broken record was now playing in my mind and it kept repeating itself, "It is NOT a cyst, it is NOT a cyst...." While trying not to listen to the words in my mind, I was also trying not to cry. I was swallowing hard while continuing to try and locate something, anything for me to focus on anywhere on the ceiling. It took everything I had to do this, yet I was still not successful. I had not burst into tears, but I had to keep blinking my tears away. The two women were either totally unaware that I was upset, or they chose not to react to it. But, by now, tears were streaming down my face.

The doctor explained that she would give me a stronger anesthetic, because she would perform a needle biopsy to take some tissue samples. These would then be sent to the lab, examined, then the results sent to my family doctor. She waited a few minutes for the anesthetics to take effect before she inserted a much larger needle. She told me I would hear a sound like a gun, and not to worry about this, that the sound was the worst part and it would not hurt much. But even with the added freezing, this needle hurt—a lot! I spoke softly, so I would not make them angry with me again, and told the two women that it hurt. One of them gave me a little more local anesthetic, but it still hurt! Imagine sticking a pin into your breast and pulling it back out.

I began to count: I had been told they would take five separate tissue samples.

I counted down.

One was already down.

That meant four to go....

I heard the sound of the gun and felt the immediate pain.

Two.

Three to go....

Not even half way there.

How long would this take?

There, the sound of the gun; instantly, the searing pain.

Three.

Two to go....

It was so painful was it almost over?

Time had slowed down again—surely it had not taken as much time as it felt it had? Finally, the last sample was taken; this latest ordeal was over. I had been so tense that now I could relax a little. I was bandaged up and given a prescription for painkillers. I was told to get dressed and I was dismissed. This time, I left without hearing the reassuring words that it was probably a cyst. Now they, too, knew what I had known from the moment that I had felt it, that this lump was NOT a cyst.

After I walked out of the Mall, I drove toward Ieke's friend's office to pick up Ieke. She looked great and came toward me to give me a hug. I flinched a little at the thought of anything close to my breast. The freezing was wearing off and the spot where the tissue had been taken was beginning to throb with pulsing pain. Ieke could sense my reluctance and, since she knew where I had been, she gave me a very gentle barely-there-hug. The years fell away. Immediately we fell into the easy conversation, which has always been our friendship's trademark. The three of us talked for a few minutes, and then Ieke and I left so Ieke's friend could return to work. Ieke and I talked and talked; we talked the entire way home. We were trying to bridge seven years, not needing to, because they fell away as if we had just spoken the day before. Ours is a "forever friendship that distance and time cannot diminish.

We did speak very briefly about the biopsy, almost dismissing it with words like "It will be fine." It was as if neither one of us wanted to admit the possibility I might not be fine. The visit was healing, comforting, and nurturing for me. We had six wonderful days together. We laughed, we cried, we were silly, and we spoke of matters of the heart and soul. The years apart no longer existed; they had been erased. I realized how much I had missed my dear friend. She visited other people and places, during the pauses in our conversations, but they only fueled us with more topics. Time played its trick again. For a few short days, hours passed too quickly, and my fears and worries about the lump in my breast were shifted to the backburner, while in the present I had a great visit with my friend.

Far too soon, it was time for her to leave again. Saying farewell was made easy with the knowledge that in July she would return with her family and I would see her again soon. Neither of us realized how much would happen in that short time.

After what had happened previously, when I was trying to find out the date and time of my appointment, I decided that this time I would not call them at all; instead, I reasoned I would just go on with my life. However, the next day, Tuesday, May 28, I could no longer suppress the need to know, so from work I phoned and made an appointment for Wednesday. I had to find out, with certainty, one way or another what it was that was growing inside my breast.

When I came home from work, there was a message on my answering machine. It asked me to call my doctor's office and to make an appointment with my doctor about the results of the biopsy. I laughed a dry laugh; I had already made the appointment myself in the morning.

Later that day, I was driving in my car when in my mind's eye I saw myself in my doctor's office talking to her and getting the results of the biopsy. With it came an instinctive knowing that the news she gave me was ominous! It would not be long now before I would have factual information about what was growing inside my breast. And that it was growing was undeniably clear. I often checked, and it was now noticeably larger than when I had first discovered it....

Chapter Four

It is Cancer!; PLOM

Wednesday morning, May 29. Irene and Cathy and I had to be at a meeting for the city for all the Before and After School Care Programs before I had to go to my doctor's appointment. It would last all morning and we planned to go for lunch together after it was finished. My appointment with my doctor was for 11:30. I told both of them that I would quickly go to my doctor's office to get the results and then would meet them. I turned to Cathy and said, jokingly, "But if I get bad news I won't meet you: I'll probably just drive around in circles." Cathy and I normally used humor to interact with each other, but this time she did not respond in kind. She looked at me quite seriously, and her answer reflected the look on her face: "That's when you have to come!" she insisted.

At this point in our lives, I was not particularly close to my co-workers since, I had only started working for the company 6 months earlier. We were professional acquaintances, but I would remember her words only a short time later. It was the beginning of allowing myself to be supported by other people.

I arrived at my doctor's office on time, but again I had to wait. After I had waited 20 minutes and my name had still not been called, I decided to become assertive. I walked past the receptionist to the back where my doctor's nurse was sitting and told her that I had to be somewhere at 12. I was beginning to speak up for myself. The nurse did not argue with me, as I has expected; instead, she immediately walked me to an examining room. She was far more serious than normal and without her usual smile. She also did not make eye contact with me. I had not been in the examination room long (in fact I was still standing looking at a wall chart) when my doctor walked in. I turned to face her and smiled in greeting but she did not smile back; she looked upset. She asked me how I was. My smile now frozen on my face I answered, "I don't know, why don't you tell me?" At that point tears appeared into her eyes, and we both sat down. I was acutely aware of the grave look on her face. She looked seriously distressed. I wanted to blurt out, "Tell me, tell me, what it is." Instead, I waited, but it was not very long, and then she sighed deeply before she said: "I have bad news." The tears I had kept at bay for so long now came and I began to cry. I still had not heard her say the words, but she was telling me that she had bad news - surely that meant what I thought it did. And I felt that my doctor was finally confirming what I had instinctively known from the start.

But I had to hear the words. I thought to myself, "What does she mean by bad news? Maybe she means that I will be lopsided for life, that I have lopsided breasts, or something like that." It's amazing the kinds of thoughts that go through our minds at moments like this. I stopped crying for a moment and looked at her squarely and asked her directly what she meant by "bad" news. I wanted her to be specific; I needed to hear her say the words. I had to know! She only partially said them, but the message was clear. Words indelibly engraved on my psyche. She said solemnly, "They found cancer cells!" She did not say, "You have cancer," but the meaning was the same, "They had found cancer cells in the lump in my breast." I had breast cancer.

Anyone who has ever heard those words, knows what it means to have the rug pulled from under you. I began to cry again, but through my tears I stated emphatically to my doctor, "I'm not going to die!" She replied kindly, "Of course not," and my doctor cried with me! This doctor, my own doctor, was not afraid to show me her humanity. While tears continued to roll down my face I affirmed insistently more to myself than to my doctor, "I'm going to live until I'm 90!" I know that my doctor also told me other things, but I don't remember any of them.

She must have known that my ability to take in information was hindered because she passed me a piece of paper with important information on it. It gave the surgeon's name and the date of my appointment with her—it was June 5th. June 5th was the day after my mother's birthday, except my mother was no longer alive. So where do you go when you have been told that you have one of the most dreaded diseases? When who you need most is your mother? I wanted to go to my childhood home to see my Mommy, to be held and told it was all going to be OK. But that home no longer existed. I now desperately needed human comfort and I didn't know what to do....

Just then, right on cue, inside my head, I "heard" Cathy's words, "That's when you have to come!" At a time when I didn't know what to do, her words guided me into action, and I knew that I would meet Irene and Cathy as planned—but first I had to go home. My home is only two minutes away from the doctor's office and, when I got home, I phoned Pa. He must have been waiting by the phone because he picked it up after the first ring. When I heard his voice, I choked; I could hardly speak, but somehow I managed through my tears to tell him that the lump in my breast was cancer! He was very quiet upon hearing this, but his reply was full of concern, and he offered to come over right away. His response nurtured me, and I calmed down a little and told him that I would go and meet Irene and Cathy as planned, and I would see him later. I also still had to go to one of my four part-time jobs this one was at Sylvan Learning Center, where I taught in the afternoon and evenings.

I drove in a daze to the restaurant. I kept hearing in my mind the words my doctor had spoken, "They found cancer cells...they found cancer cells...." The world around me had not changed, but in my world, everything had! I arrived late at our meeting place, where we had agreed to meet outside in the parking lot. From a distance I could see Irene and Cathy standing in front of the restaurant. I got out of the car and started walking toward them. This time I did not make eye contact, but kept my head down until I was close to them, then I looked up and burst into tears again while I choked out the words from inside my head, "They found cancer cells!"

Both women, who are normally very lively and animated, quietly hugged me and the three of us stood there silently. Upon hearing this news, they had no words. We, who normally never had any quiet moments between us, just stood soundless in that parking lot. Very subdued, we walked inside the restaurant to get lunch. I could not eat. I, who had used food as a solace for so long, could not find comfort in food for this. The thought of food was now almost repulsive to me, but to be sociable, I ordered a plate of ginger beef and surprisingly did manage to eat some of it. It could have been cardboard for all the flavor I could taste: I had to push it down my throat, where an emotional lump had formed.

After lunch, I drove home and somehow managed to get through the afternoon. I probably watched my soap opera very aptly named *Another World*. By watching TV, I was literally trying to enter another world, anything to not have to face my world, but of course I was not successful. At three o'clock, it was time to go to Sylvan Learning Center. It had occurred to me to cancel, but I knew this was a busy time and we did not have any substitute teachers, so I drove to work. When I arrived, I asked Debbie, the Director, if I could speak to her alone. I closed her office door and told her what my doctor had told me earlier that day. She was very shocked, and like everyone else did not know what to say to me. We, too, just sat there quietly for a few minutes, and then she told me that if I could work the first two hours she would cover me for the last. At the time, I thought that I could work all three, but after the first two hours I was very glad not to have to work any more. I was beginning to feel drained of strength and energy. But there was still something extremely difficult ahead of me: I had to tell my son....

I drove to my friend Heather's home where Vincent had gone after school. I had phoned her earlier to give her the news and asked her not to tell Vincent anything: I wanted to do this myself. I knew that the news would spread like wildfire through the family grapevine, and I wanted to reach him before the information did. I walked into her house, and she waited until Vincent was out of sight before she gave me a silent heartfelt hug. I could see in her eyes that the news had touched her deeply. She, usually also not at a loss for words, was silent after hearing this news. I had suspected earlier, when I wanted to blurt out to people that I had found a lump in my breast, that people would be shocked. I had not realized the silence this news would be met with.

I called Vincent, and together we walked outside, side by side, into my friend's garden. I was trying to find the "right" words to tell my son the news that his only parent was diagnosed with breast cancer. How do you give your child that information? I didn't know. This is the time when there should have been another parent to help buffer him from this shocking news and be strong for him. But there was no other parent; I was his sole parent. I was not only the nurturer, but also the strong one, the one who was always there for him, to help him, to guide him, to comfort and nurture him. I did not know how to support him; how could I help him with this? I was still trying to think of the right words to tell him, when just then my oldest sister Marian walked towards us. She had driven more than an hour to be with us. She also hugged me, and for a minute I cried a little, while telling her in Dutch that I had not yet told Vincent.

Whatever had felt difficult before was nothing compared to what I was feeling now. I was feeling so powerless at the thought of having to give my son this devastating news. This had to be one of the most difficult things a parent ever has to do. How can you possibly tell your child that you have been diagnosed with and are about to fight a deadly disease? What words do you use knowing that those words would crush his world, that it would mean the end of innocence for him? He was only 14 years old, still so young, only at the threshold of maturity. How do you tell your child, whose only parent you are, that you have cancer? Marian, who had been present at his

41

birth, asked if I wanted her to tell him. I said no. I knew that he had to hear it from me. Marian said that she was coming home with me and that Pa was on his way to my house and would meet us there. This was very comforting. We all walked to our cars. I was still thinking about how to tell Vincent as we stepped into the car.

As soon as Vincent and I were in the car, he looked straight at me, and before I had a chance to say anything to him, he blurted out in his customary forthright manner, "So what's the news? You got your results today, didn't you?" It was not a time for holding back and trying to cushion the information. Kind honesty was required now, and in response to his blunt question, I nodded and quietly explained to him that it was not good news, and then I told him that they had found cancer cells. He took the news stoically, briefly looked away but promptly returned his clear bright blue-eyed gaze to me and stated emphatically, in a manner similar to how I had earlier spoken in the doctor's office, "Well you're not going to die, because you have to see my grandchildren!" We smiled lopsided smiles at each other, and I answered him that, of course, I would not die, and that, yes, I would see his grandchildren. Was this a slip of the tongue and did he mean my grandchildren, or would I really live to see his grandchildren, my great-grandchildren? Both thoughts were very comforting to me. I don't remember much of the rest of the evening, other than that Pa met us at our home. We all drank coffee and just sat together for a while. I felt thankful for Pa and my sister's presence. They did not stay for a long time because I was beginning to feel total exhaustion. I wanted to rest, to go to sleep, but I wondered whether I would be able to sleep.

I did sleep that night, but I had many sleepless nights ahead of me. I know I must have worked the Thursday that followed, but I don't remember anything about that day, at all. I was in a daze. But on Friday, at the office, surrounded by my co-workers, the daze I had been in wore off and I began to go into shock. I could barely speak, or even move, let alone think. It was as if my body was beginning to shut down, one function after the other. Irene asked whether I had eaten anything, yet. I had not been able to, so she took control and insisted that I go with her and we would have something to eat. I meekly followed her, incapable of making any decision of my own, as the two of us walked over to Subway. There, looking at food, I felt that I would never be able to swallow another bite ever again. But Irene insisted that I had to eat something. The act of deciding what to eat felt like a momentous task, a task I almost felt incapable of completing, but one Irene helped me with. She made all the decisions for me. She suggested I eat a small bun with tuna and drink some juice. I was very grateful that she was making choices for me and was in charge. Everything felt like a huge effort. When our food arrived, I was surprised that I was able to swallow something, after all. But Irene recognized that I needed to get home soon, before I would not be able to drive my car, at all. All my senses were shutting down. This was my body's way of dealing with severe stress.

Somehow I made it to my house, but home was a very forlorn place. Everyone, after having initially phoned, was processing this news their own way. I was now left alone. The news had initially been met with silence, but now the quiet of my home was deafening. The phone remained silent, the doorbell did not ring, and I was beginning to slide into an abyss of self pity. I moved lethargically and robotically through the rest of Friday, all of Saturday, and Sunday morning. I was feeling alone and abandoned. I don't remember talking to Vincent or doing anything of consequence that weekend.

Forgotten were the words I had said to my doctor in her office, emphatically telling her that I was not going to die, that I would live to be 90 years old. I was lying on the couch, feeling very sorry for myself now, convinced that I was going to die! I was drowning in self-pity. The lack of human contact was taking its toll. I had a serious case of 'PLOM' disease, Poor Little Old Me! I was alone with my doubts, fears and drenched in un-supportive emotions.

Chapter Five

Row, Row, Row My Boat!

Shortly after 12 noon on Sunday afternoon, breaking through the silence, startling me in my silent home, the phone rang. It was Irene, my co-worker. She asked me if I would like it if she came over for tea. I grasped at the chance to see another human being—anyone would do. No one else, since Pa and Marian the first day, Wednesday, had asked to just come and be with me. Thursday and Friday had been spent in shock and I had been able to fill my days largely with work related items. But the weekend had arrived and everything seemed to have stopped. The silence and lack of human interactions were seriously affecting my state of mind, my state of emotions, and had increased my fear to a dangerous level so that I was now "dying" on the couch. Irene and I were, at that time, co-workers and acquaintances—we had not yet become friends. But she was a person, and I desperately needed human contact.

Irene lives almost an hour's drive away from me, on the other side of the city. While waiting for her, I continued to feel sorry for myself and to lie on the couch, "dying." After all, I had just been given a death sentence, hadn't I? In my mind's eye I saw how the visit would be. We would sit on the couch together and have tea. Our faces would be cheerless and show the distress we were feeling; after all, my situation was very sad. We would talk with our heads lowered and our voices hushed and muted. In my mind, I continued to play out the scenario. We would just sit quietly for a while drinking our tea and, after that, Irene would leave. That is how I envisioned the entire visit in my mind's eye.

Promptly after an hour had passed, Irene arrived. She rang the doorbell. I, dragging my feet, walked slowly, as if greatly aged, to the door and, subdued, opened it. Irene was barely inside, when she suggested that we go back outside. Irene knew that I live close to a lake and have lake privileges, so she asked about the lake. "Why don't we go there?" she suggested. "We could just sit on a bench." I had only recently moved to the area and I had not been to the lake yet. As a result, I did not know how it all operated. Somewhat reluctantly, I agreed, although a part of me just wanted to run through the previously imagined scenario, sitting on my couch together with Irene, feeling sorry for me. Although the lake is walking distance from my home, we got into Irene's car and drove to it. After we walked through the gate, we found a bench overlooking the water, where we sat down.

Our conversation was subdued when we first sat. We talked a little about how I was feeling, but we mostly avoided the "C" word. Except for the fact that we were not on my couch having tea, this part was very much how I had imagined it in my head earlier. The day was sunny, and it was actually pleasant to be sitting by the water, and I began to relax a little. Since I had greatly 'aged' from my PLOM disease, we sat there like two sedate middle-aged matrons.

I'm not exactly sure when it happened, but something in my mood slowly began to change. It may have started when Irene and I, at about the same time, became aware that people were getting in and out of little rowboats. They seemed to be having a good time; as a result of watching their enjoyment, my energy began to change: it began to rise a little. Irene turned to me and asked if we could use the boats too and if we had to pay for it. I told her I didn't know because this was my first visit to the lake. "Why don't we go and ask?" she suggested. I didn't really want to get off the bench and away from my self-pity; nevertheless,

I thought "Oh, well, why not?" We got up and strolled to the booth at the entrance of the lake to ask if we could use the small rowboats and how much it would cost. The attendant told us that we could and that it would not cost us anything—all we had to do was leave my lake identification card with him and, in return, he would give us oars and lifejackets. We each took a life jacket and an oar and started walking towards the boats. We felt ready to step into a rowboat and start rowing on the lake.

Our walk to the attendant had been slow, but our walk away from him had more spring to it. We now had a purpose. I was beginning to feel a little excited. Both of us were giggling a little when we, in true landlubber's fashion, put our lifejackets on. While we balanced our oars, we carefully stepped into one of the little boats. It wobbled a bit, but we managed to sit down together on the middle seat. We each put our oar into a holder, and there we sat, feeling like proud sailors, side by side on the middle bench, each one of us eagerly holding our oar. We were ready to row. I undid the lock, which held the boat attached to the shore. We were now off, or so we thought. This was a little easier said than done. Both of us, with our individual oars, gave it a good effort, as we sat together on that middle bench. We dipped our oars into the water in such a way we thought rowing should be done. But our boat did not budge: something had to be wrong; our boat did not want to move away from the shore.

We were not gliding smoothly and effortlessly, like the other rowboats, away from the shore. In fact we were not moving, at all. I looked over at one of the other boats moving smoothly across the lake, I noticed that this man was not sitting like we were. "Irene," I said, "look at that man: he is facing the other way." Well, we were willing to try anything, so both of us stood up at the same time so we could turn around and face the other way. This made our little boat rock quite dangerously. We immediately sat down, and then tried again. This time we coordinated ourselves better; first, Irene changed direction, then I did. We still had not moved away from where our little boat had been moored. It was as if we were still attached to the chain, bound to shore, even though we had unfastened the lock.

We both tried moving our oars again; still nothing happened. What were we doing wrong? Again, I looked over to the other boat gliding effortlessly across the lake. "Irene," I said, "that man is sitting alone; maybe we should do that, too." She looked, too, and sure enough, the man in the other boat was sitting alone on the middle bench. His passenger was sitting across from him, facing him. Well, maybe we should try that, too. Again, both of us stood up very enthusiastically to let the other sit on the bench alone. This, again, made our little boat rock.

By now, we were no longer giggling softly: we were laughing out loud. The harder the boat rocked, the harder we laughed. We could not even stand up because we were now laughing so hard. It was difficult to keep our balance. Finally, after much laughter, and when we had calmed down somewhat, we were ready to try again. This time, we were definitely more coordinated. We also had a plan. Irene would move to the bench at the rear of the boat, I would stay on the middle bench, and then I was going to row us out of the dock, around the lake, smoothly and effortlessly. I placed the oars in the water the way I had watched the man in the other boat do. And this time, there was some movement, and it looked like we were finally going to leave the shore behind us. It had only taken us 15-20 minutes, so far. Now that we were finally moving, I thought, how hard can this be: I would row us to the end of the lake and back. There was only a slight obstacle standing in our way: I could not seem to stop the boat from moving around in a circle. Watching our boat go around in a circle only made us laugh more hysterically, and this stopped it from moving again. By now, everything had become funny; we just could not stop laughing. Much of the tension I had stored up from the events preceding was being laughed away.

We had left the dock, but we were still very close to the shore. We were certainly not moving any great distances, nor were we anywhere close to gliding smoothly and effortlessly across the lake. Again, I tried to move my oars into the water by trying to copy the movements the man in the other boat was making. Why did our boat not progress effortlessly across the water as his boat did? His boat moved; ours only kept going around in circles. We were now laughing so hard that our boat seemed to be permanently rocking. "Let me try," Irene said. "Sure," I answered. Forgotten was our previously choreographed plan, as both of us stood up at the same time, rocking the boat more and laughing even harder. Anyone watching us must have questioned our sanity or sobriety. We managed to change position after all, but Irene did not fare any better than I did. All in all, we had now been on the water for almost an hour, yet had not strayed more than a few meters from shore.

The little boat may not have been moving much, but something else was—something was happening to my state of mind. I'm not sure of the exact moment in that little boat when I decided I was not going to die—I was going to live! Not only was I going to live, I was going to fight this disease with all I had. No longer did I want to return to my couch to continue dying: I was going to do all I could to live! My friend Jenni had phoned before the weekend and told me that during a visit to our chiropractor he had urged her to tell me to come and see him because he had some information he wanted to give me. During my earlier "dying" moments, I had not thought that I would do this; now I knew I would go and see him the next day.

Irene and I finally decided to forego our attempts at rowing effortlessly and smoothly across the lake, and amidst great laughter, were somehow able to return the little boat the short distance to the shore. Not without some exertion but certainly with great merriment, we re-attached our little vessel to its lock and returned our oars and lifejackets. Irene's visit had given me more than she and I realized at that time. It had changed my attitude—I was no longer accepting death. I was now embracing life!

I also knew that I would go and see my chiropractor, Dr. Jones, as soon as possible. I was not sure what good it would do, but it was a starting point. Years earlier, I had suffered from a herniated disc. I had been in great distress and suffered lots of pain. Initially, I had traveled the road prescribed by the "mainstream" medical community. It had been a long, hard road, filled with pain. After about six weeks of agony, the pain began to subside: a few more weeks of tolerable pain before I was finally pain free again and could move with some ease. I probably had only two pain free weeks before I fell on a piece of ice and hurt my back again, this time worse than before, and the doctor I was seeing started mentioning surgery. I did not want surgery, so I started looking for an alternative treatment and, on the recommendation of a friend, I "found" Dr. Jones.

The difference between my first attack with the herniated disc, doing what "mainstream" medicine deemed necessary and being treated by Dr. Jones, chiropractor, was startling, to say the least. Not only was my recovery time noticeably less, but the fact that I recovered without need for surgery helped build a deep trust I feel for Dr. Jones. Over the years, I would have increasingly smaller episodes of back pain, and always found relief from my visits to Dr. Jones. Since that time, I now see him once a month for maintenance to keep my back strong.

I was not sure what a chiropractor could offer me in a battle against cancer, but in the past he had always been brutally honest, and over the years we had some interesting discussions about the analysis of illnesses and their origins. So when I went to see Dr. Jones the next day, Monday, I was not sure what he could offer me, if anything; but since my shift in consciousness after rowing with Irene, I was more open and willing to go and find out.

Chapter Six

Hope!

SEEING DR. JONES

Monday afternoon, I drove the short distance to Dr. Jones' office. The visit started as it always had. My heightened senses were more acutely aware of the differences between his office and the mainstream medical community. I was met by a smile from Debbie, who was sitting at the receptionist desk, as she greeted me by name; I was not a number here. The waiting room was clean, uncluttered, and filled with current and interesting magazines; however, before I could begin to read any of them I was taken into an examination room. This room was bright and airy, and a healthy looking living plant was trying to push against the ceiling. On the wall was a white quote board where Dr. Jones or one of his assistants writes sayings. The saying for that day was, "Yesterday has already passed, tomorrow is still a dream, but today is here, that is why it is called 'The Present'."

I could feel myself begin to relax. I realized how tense I had been. It was less than five minutes when Dr. Jones walked into the room. His smile felt warm and sincere, but I could see concern in his eyes as well. Jenni had spoken to him about my diagnosis, so I knew that he was aware of what I was facing.

"You heard from Jenni that I have breast cancer, right?" I jumped right in.

He nodded.

"She said I should come and see you."

"Yes," he replied, "because I want to offer you any support I can."

"What can you do? You are a chiropractor, not a cancer specialist?"

"Yes, that is true, but it is important that you support your body during this difficult time. Remember when you first came here, years ago, and I explained to you then that chiropractic treatments neither treat any symptoms, nor cures any disease? Chiropractic treatments locate and correct spinal nerve interference and let the body heal itself. Keeping the spine and nervous system healthy helps the immune system stay strong. With what you're facing and with whatever form of treatment you decide to take, try as much as possible to strengthen and support your immune system."

"But how do I do that?" I asked. I was confused; he made it sound as if I had a choice and it also sounded as if I could do things to help myself—could that be true, or was I misreading his message?" As if he had read my mind, he continued.

"You have been diagnosed with cancer, but you are not helpless, there is a lot you can do to support yourself. Become an active participant in your process!!" He paused a few seconds to allow me to process this statement before he continued. "Chiropractic treatments, exercise, nutrition, laughter, controlling the stress response all help to boost your immune system," he said, then added,

"The first thing I would recommend that you do is to read all you can about cancer. Find out what cancer is, go to the public library and the University library and do your own research. Learn all you can about this condition, become informed, read as much as you can about breast cancer and what the latest treatments are; learn about possible causes, talk to and read about other women who have been treated."

I was a little taken back by the amount of information he was trying to give me, but as he continued talking, I began to get a sense that having breast cancer might not automatically mean a death sentence. "You mean to say," I asked, "that having breast cancer does not necessarily mean that I will die?"

"Lots of people recover from cancer and there is a lot you can do to prepare yourself for the tough road ahead. What kind of treatment are they recommending for you?" he asked.

"I don't know yet," I replied. "I'm meeting with a surgeon on Wednesday, the 5th of June." Today was June third.

"That gives you an entire day to become more informed." He said.

"I hope you don't mind, but I asked my assistant to photocopy you some material I have on breast cancer and also information on what you can do to strengthen your immune system. Are you interested in reading this material?"

I nodded eagerly. I was not only interested, but felt an immense need to learn more about the danger that I was facing with this illness called cancer.

"Information is your friend," Dr. Jones continued; "gather as much of it as you can. I also believe that the cancer clinic has a library where patients can borrow books. I recommend that you go and take advantage of that library, too. And don't forget to ask lots of questions from the doctors you have to see. Take someone with you and write the questions down before you see them; then, when you are there, have the person who is with you write the answers down, so you won't forget them. "

Next, he started to explain how cancer cells get started and our body's role in this process. He drew me a picture of healthy cells to help me grasp the cellular process. To make it easy for me to understand, he drew the healthy cells as squares with a dot in the middle. He explained that every cell gets replaced and that in a healthy body, healthy cells replace healthy cells. So far that was easy to understand. I had learned that in my High School Biology class. Then he continued the explanation by telling me that when our body is exposed to stress or our immune system is weakened, the cells begin to change. At first, a little change takes place, after which the squares don't quite look square anymore: The edges become softer. I asked him to repeat this, so I could more fully understand.

He did, and then he resumed by adding that if nothing gets done to stop the square cells from correcting themselves, the change continues and the square cells begin to change shapes even more. He drew arrows between the changing shapes to help me understand. The last shape was no longer square at all. Now, the "cells" had totally changed and were the shape of a triangle.

"This is what happens when people are ill and have a disease," he explained. But I noticed that he wrote the word "disease" differently. He wrote it not as one word but as two separate words: Dis Ease! He explained that Dis Ease means that the body is *not* at ease and that there is a lot we can do to bring our bodies back to a state of Ease.

It sort of made sense to me what he was saying, but I had a hard time keeping my focus. The fear and shock I was feeling over having been diagnosed with cancer were hindering my ability to fully understand what he was saying. I felt like I was listening through a fog. But Dr. Jones was patient and gave me the information in its simplest form. Even then, it would take time before I fully understood what he was saying. But in time, I got it. What he said sounded logical and encouraging. Yes, I was going to do my research and read as much as I could about breast cancer. I was also eager to see the articles his assistant had copied for me. I agreed to come back and see him again in a few days, after my appointment with the surgeon.

He gave me a chiropractic treatment before I left and mentioned another treatment he would start me on when I came back in a few days. It was called M. E. S. or *Microcurrent Electrical Stimulation*. He explained that the theory behind this method is that there is a direct-current electrical system present in our bodies. This electrical system is responsible for keeping our tissues healthy. When our bodies are injured there is a shift in the normal current flow and balance, and the electrical current is no longer flowing as it should. Dr. Jones explained that M. E. S. mimics the body's natural frequency and, by doing so, facilitates healing and recovery. My body was not necessarily injured but because of my weakened immune system the electrical current was also not functioning as it should have.

"Will it be painful?" I asked

"No," he answered. "The current is so small that most likely you will not feel anything at all. It is not like the other tingly electrotherapy for treatment of back muscles,"

I still didn't really understand it all clearly because there was so much information and so much was happening to me, but somehow it sounded logical and I was willing to give it a try. I also knew that Dr. Jones believes in non-toxic, non-invasive healing methods. This knowledge reassured me that whatever information and suggestions he would offer me would do no harm. The treatments he had given me in the past had never caused me any harm and had only been beneficial, so I had no reason to feel that it would be any different now.

When I left his office, I had a large envelope filled with articles firmly clutched under my arm. I was very curious what I would discover.

Chapter Seven

Learning about Cancer

INFORMATION

As soon as I got home, I eagerly began to read the information Dr. Jones had given me. I was astonished, amazed and shocked by what I was reading. Several articles I read were from a magazine called *Health & Healing—Tomorrow's Medicine Today*. The first article I read was written by an M. D. named Julian Whitaker. The article was called "What I Would Do If I Had Cancer." I was very curious to read what a doctor would do if he were diagnosed with cancer. The first sentence I read shocked me because it stated, "We are obviously losing ground with conventional cancer treatment because the death rates for cancer keep going up." Well, he got my attention. I eagerly resumed reading and he continued by saying that what he called conventional treatments are based on a paradigm. This model is based on the belief that we have to purge the body of cancer by using aggressive and toxic methods such as surgery, chemotherapy, and radiation therapy.

He continued to say that statistics do not tell the real story and that these statistics do not tell how people died. With astonishment, I read the following statement, "Conventional therapy is so toxic and dehumanizing that I fear it far more than I fear death from cancer." I was completely hooked now; I had to find out why he felt that way and, more importantly, I wanted to find out if there was another way to fight cancer.

I, like most people, had always thought that there was only one way to battle the disease and that was to have surgery or chemotherapy or radiation therapy or any combination of these three treatments. I sensed from the beginning of this article that this doctor knew something I did not yet know: That there was another way to fight cancer.

Dr. Whitaker wrote that we know that conventional therapy does not work and that if conventional therapy works we would not fear cancer anymore than we fear pneumonia. I had never given it much thought, but as I read it, I had to agree with what he was saying. I knew the fear I had already encountered from my family and friends and in myself. I had suffered with pneumonia in the past and telling people about that illness had been a very different experience.

With fascination, I read about people with cancer who tried to find the so called alternative methods and how these methods were treated by the *FDA* (*Food and Drug Administration*). Dr. Whitaker mentioned two clinics that had been hounded for years by the *FDA*. This man had done his research; this was not a hocus pocus little article. It told the story of a doctor who uses Immune Augmentative Therapy (IAT) which was started in the mid-1960's and showed success; however, when he tried to get *FDA* approval it became very clear that the *FDA* appeared to be far more interested in blocking his way instead of facilitating the process, so he moved his clinic to the Bahamas.

The other clinic mentioned told a comparable story, again about a so called alternative treatment which had also shown success and had received an almost identical treatment from the *FDA*. This clinic is located in Texas. It also said that other countries appear to be more open and are looking into licensing these treatments. I wanted to read more, but I made a mental note to myself that I would phone Ieke and find out what was happening in the Netherlands in the form of cancer treatment and alternative treatments. Maybe she could send me Dutch information and I could continue to educate myself. I went back to the second page of the article where Dr. Whitaker was writing about an imaginary scenario where he had cancer and what he would do if this were true.

I was very curious to find out what an alternative minded M. D. would do if he had cancer. First he wrote that he wanted to make it very clear that whatever a person chooses, it is a personal choice based on an individual belief system. As I read it, I realized that this echoed Dr. Jones' approach.

There was one sentence which really leaped out at me. It said, "Because we are strongly influenced by our natural fear of death, we line up for conventional cancer therapy, not so much believing that it will work, but hoping it will not fail." I stopped reading for a moment to really absorb that statement. I felt in my deepest knowing that this was so true. I thought back to the night when I had discovered the lump. Feeling the hardening knob under my skin had instantly jolted me to a place of deep fear based on cancer and death. That night I was reminded of my own mortality and the possibility that I could die. Remembering that I knew that most people are so afraid of death that they will do just about anything to stop it from happening, and I was not any different. And yet, I also knew that death is one of life's certainties: It will happen to all of us. I knew that some day it would certainly happen to me too; however, I was determined that this was not the time. A strong knowing grew inside me that this cancer was not a death sentence for me.

Dr. Whitaker went on with his imaginary cancer scenario. The first few paragraphs were filled with what he would NOT do, but more importantly he added why: He wrote that he would NOT even check in with a conventional oncologist. At this point in my reading, I have to admit that I did not even know what an oncologist was (a specialist in tumors), so I did not really absorb the significance of this statement. But his reason for not doing so made sense based on what I had already read. He said that oncologists are used to implementing the erroneous paradigm that cancer must be purged from the body with toxic methods. He compared that to having maps for a flat earth.

I continued reading, and he said that he would NOT take

a passive role. That I could understand. The previous day, after my rowing adventure with Irene, I had felt a strong urging to take action, to do something. I did not want to take a passive approach and my visit with Dr. Jones, including the material I was now reading, had only validated this. Dr. Whitaker continued to say that taking a passive role with today's conventional methods is terribly dangerous, because the drugs alone could easily cause death—and he emphasized, this would not be unusual. I read with alarmed fascination that there are numerous cases of iatrogenic (doctor induced) deaths from chemotherapy. Somewhere, faraway sounding, a phone rang, but I was too absorbed to answer it. I could not stop; I had to keep reading this eye-opening material to find out more.

I nodded with agreement as Dr. Whitaker stated he would actively fight for his life, because I too was feeling very strongly that I wanted to actively fight for mine! He mentioned the two clinics again and how he would use their treatments, but not just that: He validated what Dr. Jones had told me earlier that day, that he would head to the public library to make a battle plan. The last sentence of this paragraph was disturbing— Patients who seek alternative treatments are more optimistic and they have only one worry—the cancer, not the cancer *and* the therapy!

Wow, that was certainly a strong statement to make. Could any of this be true? It sounded like a conspiracy from *FDA* agencies against people who were trying something different. And was it really true that the conventional treatments did not work or had such a low success rate? I had to find out more. I realized that what I was reading was one person's opinion. From my University days and the research I had done for different courses, I knew that I had to find different sources to get to a stronger measure of truth. But I was not yet done with this article, so I continued reading with increased fascination.

What more would this doctor tell me? I read on. What would he do? And there it was again: He said that he would turn his back on 50 years of institutionalized expertise because he felt that they were following the wrong paradigm. And then he wrote how he viewed cancer and which paradigm he would use, "Cancer is a systemic problem in which the normal control mechanisms of your body are altered. Your immune system likely bears the largest burden for this control; thus, all techniques that enhance it are promising. Those that damage it are not!" I stopped reading again to let this information sink in, to really absorb what I was reading.

I read the passage again. Since I was under stress, it still felt like I was seeing, hearing, and understanding through a fog; it was difficult to totally grasp it. I had read somewhere that when people are faced with stress, their ability to understand drops dramatically. Well, mine certainly had. I wanted to understand what he said here, but I was having a hard time doing it. What I did understand from it is the importance of the immune system. I did not yet understand what he meant, but during the next weeks and months it would all become much clearer and I would remember what I read today with greater understanding.

He said that he would change his diet. He would switch to a mostly vegetarian diet and would reduce his caloric intake to about 1500, two or three times a week. His reason was that by eating fewer calories, the immune system becomes stronger and that caloric reduction also increases the levels of human growth hormones. I had no idea what hormones he was talking about, but I did understand the part about helping the immune system get stronger. I began to understand what I had read earlier, that somehow something has gone wrong in our bodies when we have cancer and that we can do something by helping our immune system get stronger. I wasn't quite sure what had gone wrong in mine, but I did understand that I could help my immune system, except I was not sure how, yet. But I was going to continue my quest for information; surely, I would discover something in the articles that would be helpful.

I realized that a battle plan was beginning to form in my mind: I would change my diet and I would try to strengthen my immune system (how I was going to do all that was not yet clear, but I had no doubt that it would become clearer from my research). Well, help and understanding were closer by than I thought. The next paragraph gave me some concrete things I could do to strengthen my immune system.

Dr. Whitaker wrote that he would take nutritional supplements and gave examples. At the time of my reading I was totally ignorant about nutritional supplements. I had held a personal belief that all the nutrients we needed we received from the foods we ate. I also believed that taking nutritional supplements were unnecessary and a waste of money. I had no idea just how uninformed I had been but over the next weeks, which were filled with more research, I began to realize just how unaware I really was.

He recommended high doses of vitamin C, between 6,000 to 10,000 mg per day. Vitamin C is a powerful antioxidant that fights free radicals (cancer cells). I decided that, in my case, more was better and since I already knew that our bodies get rid of excess vitamin C, my decision was to take 10,000 mg of timed released Vitamin C @ day. The Dr. also wrote that the Mayo Clinic had conducted two studies on Vitamin C and in both studies found that Vitamin C did not work. However, he added, that both studies were set up in a way that guaranteed failure. He did not give details as to how they did this but he added that he feels that this was done intentionally to create negative publicity for this non-toxic approach. I did not know if this was true, but I did not think that Vitamin C was something which would hurt me. So, item #1 on my battle plan - taking 10,000 mg of Vitamin C.

Next, he wrote about shark cartillage, Coenzyme Q10, and Essiac Tea. I was not sure about any of these three: I wanted to do some more research on them, so that day I did not add them on my list. Dr. Whitaker finished his article by writing that he would keep searching for effective non-toxic therapies. That would also be part of my battle plan.

I was feeling overwhelmed by what I had just read and also sensed that I might be experiencing some information overload. I stood up and stretched before I found the next article I wanted to read. This was an interview with a doctor with Questions and

Answers called: "Questioning Chemotherapy" with a statement by Dr. Ralph W. Moss PhD. I noticed the PhD. behind his name. Well, that certainly gave him credentials. He was not someone just throwing out statements. Dr. Moss said, "Chemotherapy drugs are the most toxic substances ever put deliberately into the human body." Now, that was certainly a powerful statement to make. I was not sure how much more information I could absorb, so I decided to take a break first. I made myself a cup of coffee, not realizing that it would be my last cup for a long time to come.

When I finished my coffee, I felt ready to tackle the interview with Dr. Ralph Moss. I read that Ralph Moss, PhD is recognized as one of the most knowledgeable people in the world on the subject of alternative cancer therapies. He is also a medical science writer and a former assistant director of public affairs at the Memorial Sloan-Kettering Cancer Centre. The article stated that Dr. Moss has written eight books and was the author of an award winning PBS documentary called *The Cancer War*. All of this did not mean much to me, but it did appear to indicate that Dr. Moss was indeed an authority on this topic.

Once more, what I read shocked me and opened both my eyes and mind. Dr. Moss claims that chemotherapy is only useful for a few relatively rare kinds of cancer. Then he said that for the vast majority of solid tumors in adults, chemotherapy is not only inappropriate and ineffective, it is downright dangerous as well. I read that there have been significant improvements in acute lymphocytic leukemia (ALL) , Hodgkin's disease, and testicular cancer and that, in these cases, chemotherapy is quite successful and a rational choice. What I did not see mentioned was breast cancer. I had to find out more and see if he mentioned breast cancer at all. So I continued reading and, sure enough, there, in the next paragraph, it was in black and white: "The vast majority of cancers, however, are solid tumors of adults – such as *breast*, colon, lung – and these are barely touched by chemotherapy. "

There it was: Breast cancer, according to this doctor was barely touched by chemotherapy. The interviewer asked the question that was certainly on my mind. Why then do we keep reading and hearing about progress in the use of chemotherapy in cancer? How would Dr. Moss answer this question? The answer was on the next page and with great anticipation, I turned the page. I had to read the page a few times to understand what I was reading.

Dr. Moss said that the *FDA* defines the "response" to a drug as a 28-day shrinkage of 50 per cent or more of all measurable tumors. Then he continued on to say that there is no correlation between tumor shrinkage and the extension of life. It was as if I was reading another language. Didn't we want the tumor to shrink? The interviewer must have thought the same because he asked the question and Dr. Moss answered that this is only important if a tumor is disfiguring or pressing on a nerve, causing pain. He also said that in the majority of cases shrinkage of a tumor is not of primary importance. Once more I realized how very little I actually knew about cancer and tumors. I had always assumed that the most important thing in the fight against tumors and cancer was to shrink the tumor and yet this doctor was saying that this was not necessarily the case.

There was one more question the interviewer asked, "Hasn't chemo been shown to prolong life?" The answer again was surprising because it said that there was no automatic correlation that showed that tumor shrinkage leads to increased life. Then the interviewer mentioned that Dr. Moss' position was supported by many major students of the statistics of cancer treatments and he gave some facts and names. They meant very little to me other than to give credibility to what this man was saying. The article certainly did not appear to be based on a hunch or feeling. This was a highly educated person who had done tons of research.

NOTE: More on Dr. Moss can be found on the following websites: .

1. http://www.cancerdecisions.com
2. http://www.ralphmoss.com/html/reports.shtml

The article also said that in a number of surveys most chemotherapists said that they themselves would not take the treatment, nor would they recommend it for their families.

Wow, I was more confused than ever. Here was what I believed to be one of the accepted treatments for cancer, and this doctor was saying that it was largely ineffective and certainly very dangerous. The article was only two pages long and I had come to the end of it. I rummaged through the papers given to me by Dr. Jones to see if there was anything else on chemotherapy. I could not find anything else, but my eyes had been openend, and I decided that I wanted to know more information on what chemotherapy was and how it was used in cancer treatments.

I did not feel that doing research on chemotherapy was too pressing for me that day because it would not apply to me. The first step in my treatment was to meet with the surgeon on Wednesday and schedule surgery to have the tumor removed. It was possible that the doctors would recommend chemotherapy after surgery, but I had lots of time to do research before I needed to worry about that. Surgery was first on the agenda, and I was quite certain that I would not even consider chemotherapy after that even if was offered to me.

I looked at one other article before I stopped reading for the day. These were pages from a book called *Prescription for Nutritional Healing,* by James F. Balch, M. D. and Phyllis A. Balch, CNC. This is where I discovered recommendations about what to eat and what supplements to take. It recommended drinking distilled water and lots of it to flush out the toxins, and eating onions and garlic everyday. Well, that seemed to make sense and it was do-able for me, so I added that to my list. Next, it said to eat ten raw almonds a day because they are high in laetrile which acts as an anti-cancer agent. Almonds, too, were added to my list. Then the article went on to say that all anti-cancer diets should include grains, nuts, seeds and unpolished, brown rice. I was already adding nuts in the form of almonds and would add the brown rice.

Then the article gave a list of what not to eat and I decided not to eat these for awhile, that it would be a small price to pay. It warned against junk food, processed refined foods, saturated fats, salt, sugar and white flour. It also said to eliminate alcohol, coffee, and all teas except herbal teas. It mentioned that large amounts of coffee weaken the immune system and place additional stress on the adrenal glands. I didn't know anything about adrenal glands, but I understood about weakening the immune system and from what I understood from my other readings, my immune system was already weakened, so I certainly did not want to weaken it even more. Sugar, it said, was also an immune depressor and that studies had shown that hours after consuming sugar one's immune system was still significantly lowered. That's all I needed to read to take sugar off my list of what I would consume.

It also said not to eat any animal protein and, even stronger, it recommended never eating luncheon meat, hotdogs, or smoked or cured meats because of the dangers in the nitrates used to treat the meats. It said to restrict dairy consumption because of the hormones present in dairy products. Next, it mentioned how to cook and because of potential low-level radiation leakage, to avoid microwave ovens. I could do that; I didn't use mine very much anyway, so I would for the time being just not use it all all. It also cautioned against sitting too close to television sets; it recommended sitting at least eight feet away. That was also workable, and I usually did not sit too close to the the television, anyway. Besides, it made me feel like I was actively doing something.

Then I read the importance of avoiding chemicals. The article said they promote the formation of free radicals in the body, which may lead to cancer. It also said that cancer victims will further weaken their immune system by using chemicals. The writer explained that our body has to use up energy trying to protect itself from the damaging chemicals, rather than fighting the cancer. That made sense to me. It further cautioned against the use of aerosol products for the same reasons. The chemicals the article mentioned were hair sprays, cleaning compounds, waxes, fresh paints and garden pesticides. I decided that I could certainly eliminate these products from my life and give my body the freedom to fight the cancer instead of protecting itself from these damaging chemicals. I would also not use any chemicals on my hair while the battle against cancer was raging. That meant no perms and no artificial colour treatments for my hair. I felt it was a small price to pay in order to stay alive. The one thing I would not eliminate was make-up. Although make-up was also made up of chemicals, the reason I chose to keep wearing it had to do with being a woman and wanting to look good.

I felt like I was making an important start by adding and eliminating certain foods and being aware of the effects chemicals had on my body. I decided that day that I would also elliminate foods which had been subjected to pesticides,since they fit into the chemicals mentioned, and that I would try as much as possible to only eat organic foods. I knew that I could not afford to go to the clinics mentioned in the first article because my financial situation would not allow this, but there were many other things I could do, and eliminating bad foods and chemicals, while adding good foods and nutrional supplements were, I felt, a good start.

After reading the articles, I began to see that what I had been doing to my body had been both harmful and destructive. I had not been using food as fuel: I had been slowly poisoning myself with the food I had been eating for many years. I had read that the sugar I so adored and which was so much a part of my daily intake was one of the worst culprits. I also realized how little I really knew about nutrition and what it takes to have a healthy body.

Food was one of the important aspects I read in the information laying on my kitchen table, but it was by no means all.

I further learned that cancer is a weaker cell and that in a healthy body it can easily be kept under control by our immune system. In fact, I was astonished to find out that most people form cancer cells daily and that they are just as easily destroyed by our immune system, given that our immune system works. Cancer begins to grow out of control when a person's immune system is not working properly.

The more I read, the more I became convinced that for me the answer lay in helping my immune system get strong again. From the reading, I understood that my immune system had to be severely compromised for the cancer to start growing. It then made sense to me that since this was something my body had allowed to grow, could it then also not destroy it as well, if I supported my immune system as much as I could by trying to get it back on track? It felt good to engage my mind by learning facts about cancer. It almost made me forget how afraid I was—almost....

Time had passed by unnoticed; I had been totally engrossed in the articles I was reading. They answered many questions, but also left me with more questions I wanted answers to. I wrote my questions down so I could ask the doctor I would see in a day and a half. My despair from the weekend was making place for something else: Hope! I began to understand that there were many things I could do.

That night when I went to sleep I felt better than I had for days; my visit to Dr. Jones had provided me with lots of helpful information: It was the start of my education process on the foe I was facing. But the most important thing I had received that day was Hope. I now had a sense that having breast cancer did not automatically mean a death sentence.

Chapter Eight

Rocking the Boat

The following day was Tuesday and I went into the office; there, a surprise awaited me. My boss Dan had also been busy reading and learning about cancer and he had taken a somewhat different course. In his readings he had come across information on CoenzymeQ10, Shark Cartilage, and Essiac Tea, which I had also seen in my readings. I had not found too much information in the articles I had read, but obviously he had. He had learned that taking CoenzymeQ10 was very beneficial for people with cancer, and he had bought a few bottles for me that he presented me with that day. He also gave me an information sheet on CoenzymeQ10 which said that CoenzymeQ10 had been used for "high risk" breast cancer patients. These patients had been treated with anti-oxidants and CoenzymeQ10 and that six of 21 patients showed partial tumor regression. That was encouraging for me to read, and since I had already started to incorporate anti-oxidants, I felt that taking CoenzymeQ10 as well was a good thing.

He had also read that shark cartilage helps capsulate the tumor and prevents it from growing. He explained to me how it works. As a tumor grows, it develops a network of blood vessels that provide it with the necessary blood supply and energy to survive and grow. He told me that this process is called angiogenesis. He had been very intrigued to read that Shark Cartilage is thought to prevent blood vessels from forming. The article he had read also stated that, as a result, the tumor starves because it does not get the blood and nutrients it needs. He continued by telling me that shark cartilage works best on solid tumors because these need a lot of new blood vessels to grow. This certainly included breast cancer but he said that it also included tumors of the central nervous system, cervix, prostate, and pancreas. Then he gave me a bottle of Shark Cartilage. Well, I was willing to give it a try. I took both the copy of the article he handed me and the bottle of Shark Cartilage.

But he was not finished yet. In his research he had also come across something called Essiac Tea and he was very excited to tell me about it. Once more, he had a copy of several articles for me as well as some Essiac Tea. He explained that Essiac Tea purifies your blood and that Essiac is a mixture of four herbs, Indian rhubarb, sheep head sorrel, slippery elm and burdock root. He had been very excited to read that Essiac Tea strengthens the body's immune system and so allows it to fight cancer. He continued telling me that Essiac Tea not only improves appetite, supplies vitamins, enzymes and minerals, but it also relieves pain and may prolong life. But he felt that the most important thing about Essiac Tea for me was that one of the herbs in Essiac decreases tumor growth and the others act as blood purifiers. He had read that it is beneficial for many types of cancer, including breast cancer.

I left Dan's office and went to my desk. Concentrating on work was not easy that morning. Once more I had been given lots of information, and my mind was whirling from trying to keep up with everything I was trying to process. But I also felt like I was not alone in this fight. By giving me information and products, Dr. Jones and Dan were giving me much needed support and showing me there was not just one way to look at this disease. I began to realize just how uninformed and uneducated I really was about cancer and its causes and treatments. I was now a little less afraid of my appointment the next day with the surgeon. I was eager for more information. Dan and Dr. Jones had treated me with the intelligence and support I assumed I would receive from the surgeon the next day.

Wednesday, June 5 was my appointment with the surgeon. Marian and Pa came along with me to the hospital. The adventure in the boat could have given me some clues, but until I spoke with the surgeon I did not know how much I was going to rock the boat. I had expected that she would tell me about surgery and what it would entail and when it would be. Instead she told me that she would refer me to an oncologist and that he would most likely recommend chemotherapy before surgery. Chemotherapy? I couldn't believe what I heard: Did she really mean chemotherapy? What about surgery first? I was shocked and was still processing this information, but somehow I still found my voice a little bit to reply softly to her that I thought I didn't want to do this. Perhaps I said it too quietly, or she did not wish to hear me, for she appeared to ignore what I said.

I explained that I felt that if the tumor was cut out of my breast I felt it would give me a fighting chance. I had been prepared to listen and get information; I had not been prepared for being presented with chemotherapy, especially after everything I had read two days earlier. I had at that time only been educating myself and not really made a decision to not have chemotherapy. I was not finished with my research yet.

And yet, the information I had read had left me with many questions: It had been compelling and forceful and, mostly, it appeared to say that chemotherapy was not really successful for breast cancer. I needed more information so I could make my decision based on facts. And now, here I was face to face with the fact that this woman would not perform surgery, not before I had chemotherapy. What was this? That is why I was so hesitant-sounding when I said that I did not want chemotherapy: I was not very sure yet because I had only just begun to read about it. But that day, the surgeon did not hear my not-yet-very-strong voice. And so she sent me on to the next step: to see the oncologist.

I phoned Jenni when I got home; we had only recently met but had instantly liked each other. We had a lot in common:

Both of us were under employed teachers; we were both struggling single moms; and I had taken over her job as a day home supervisor, which gave us something else in common. We had also discovered that we both had a strong spiritual yearning and were both seeking spiritual guidance and paths.

After I had read some of the articles from Doctor Jones, I had discussed them with Jenni and had voiced my concerns about the invasive methods used by traditional medicine to fight cancer. At this time, we discovered that we both had an aversion against using invasive techniques to fight an illness. I wanted to support my healing, to take an active part in it, not to give myself over to the all powerful doctors without taking an active role myself. I had just discovered there was much I could do to stimulate and support my immune system, and I was becoming more and more determined to do so.

So during this conversation after my visit with the doctor, I told Jenni about the surgeon's recommendation that I see an oncologist next and that I was to have chemotherapy first before she would even consider doing surgery. I explained to Jenni that the reasons made sense to the surgeon and were based on all she knew. The facts to the surgeon about me were: I was young, had only just turned 38, and I was pre-menopausal. This is a dangerous age to have breast cancer because I was still in my child bearing years. Because of that, the chance that the cancer would grow fast was great. Another fact was that breast cancer was present in my family and, more importantly, on my mother's side. I explained to Jenni that these were all factors which made warning bells go off for the mainstream medical community. Then there was the added fact that a maternal aunt had been diagnosed with breast cancer at 26 and had died ten years later after an agonizing awful fight against breast cancer. I had been too young to have witnessed her fight. I was only nine years old when she died, and she had lived too far away for us to visit often.

There was also the size of my tumor and the fact that it had not been there a month earlier and now it was between 1 ½" x 1 ¾" or 3 x 4 cm, easily felt by hand. Another crucial piece of information was the fact that the type of cancer they had discovered after the biopsy was an aggressive ductal cancer.

All his information strongly influenced the decisions the surgeon made and why she thought that it needed to be fought systemically. I reported to Jenni that the surgeon had explained that fighting cancer systemically was in order to make sure the cancer cells had not spread to other parts of my body. As I continued my account of the doctor's visit, I told her that I was told that they wanted to make sure that the cancer was attacked with force before the tumor would be removed by surgery. As I continued giving Jenni the details of my visit to the surgeon and what I had been told there, I told her that chemotherapy is considered a systemic treatment, which means that it reaches all parts of the body, not just the tumor and not just the cancer cells. For that reason, one of the side-effects is hair loss because chemotherapy targets all fast growing cells, and hair cells are fast growing cells.

Their reasons sounded logical, and if I had not read the articles from Dr. Jones two days earlier I would probably have consented to the procedures and their recommendations; but I had started to read and inform myself and I was not sure at all that chemotherapy was a good idea. I knew that my immune system was already very weak because that is how cancer has a chance to grow, so why would I weaken it even more by exposing myself to chemotherapy to eradicate the cancer? Yes, it was possible that chemotherapy would do this, but the articles had said that in many cases no changes were seen in the size of tumors and that it was not deemed successful for breast cancer. I was confused, and I wanted to know more. But inside me, I felt my inner voice, my inner knowing, my connection with my higher power, my connection with my soul, begin to speak, and I knew that this was the voice that knew what was best for me. I realized that the doctors I was seeing wanted the best for me, but it was based on what they knew and on what they believed in, and it did not include any information about me other than some superficial facts. They did not know what my family life was like, or who I really was, all aspects of a person I consider to be crucially important.

71

I was beginning to walk steps onto a path where I would listen to my inner wisdom and hold my own counsel. Speaking up in the surgeon's office that day was only the beginning. I would not be alone in this fight; as much as it was a solitary war, there were people waiting at the sideline, ready to support and cheer me on. Some I already knew, others would appear when I needed them.

My voice, my true self—I needed to reclaim it for the fight ahead of me and I was now determined to fight. In the surgeon's office my voice had not been sufficiently strong to be heard. The female surgeon did not or would not hear me. And I had not repeated myself. An appointment was made for me with the oncologist. I decided not to bring my dad or my sister with me. I could sense their fear for the disease and reverence to the Medical profession. I did not want to hurt them, and I did not want to argue with them. I was not yet certain whether I could be strong enough to defend myself. I was not sure how they would feel about my choice to refuse chemotherapy. It appeared that they felt I only had one choice, and that was to do what the doctors and the hospital told me. It was now becoming very clear to me that I did not want chemotherapy.

I needed someone beside me who agreed with me and supported my choice. The day of my appointment with the oncologist followed the surgeon's appointment closely. I had asked Jenni to come with me. Before this visit, I had re-read the articles Dr. Jones had given me, plus books I had picked up from the library and magazines from Health Food stores. My understanding about cancer and its treatments was deepening, just as my resolve to try the so-called alternatives was strengthened.

Going to the cancer clinic was quite an experience. A volunteer was assigned to "help" me find the area where I needed to go. I felt that this sent a message to me and my body: Cancer patients are incapable of finding where they have to go.

I decided not to fall into that mindset, the mindset of being a victim to this disease. I needed to support my feelings and thoughts with actions. So, Instead of letting the volunteer decide where I was to go, I took the lead. I did not want to take the elevator—It was only one floor down, and I headed towards the stairs. I sprinted down with purpose and with such speed that the volunteer and Jenni could barely keep up with me. I was not aware that they were behind me trying to keep pace with me. I felt that taking the elevator was another way I was giving away my power: I needed to walk, to feel alive. I had to do this for me. I needed to be strong and use my muscles, my body, not stand placidly, like an invalid, in an elevator. I had not felt sick in the days leading up to my discovery, and I did not feel sick or weak now. I did not want to think of myself as weak or sick. I did not need a volunteer to show me the way to the oncologist's office. I could find my own way. I recognize that the volunteer was well meaning, but it was not what I needed. "Needing" a volunteer to take me to the doctor's office was not the message I wanted to send to my body, to myself.

We arrived on the floor where the oncologist's office is. We had to walk down a hallway and then turn left, but before we reached his office, I received a jolt. In the corner, before we could turn left, we saw two women representing Reach to Recovery sitting behind a table showing bathing suits for women with mastectomies. I felt this was another message sent to my body, "Having Breast cancer automatically means you have to have a mastectomy." I did not wish to stop and talk to these, again, well meaning women. I did not want to buy into their belief system! I did not want my body to receive that message. I intentionally looked the other way and walked quickly past them. I'm sure that many women outwardly react the same way, based on fear. Mine was not a reaction: it was an informed purposeful response.

Jenni and I found a seat in the overflowing waiting room. While waiting for my appointment, a man walked by pushing a cart filled with coffee, tea, and cookies. He offered everyone waiting for an oncologist something to drink; no charge. This was another 'interesting' treatment for the 'poor' cancer patients. Only cancer patients and their escorts get such elitist treatment. Jenni and I did not discuss our findings in front of the other people there. It was not our intent to hurt anyone, but we discussed our views and opinions later in the car on our drive home.

My turn for the appointment arrived. My first impression of the oncologist was that of a kindly older man, with a benevolent slightly paternal bedside manner. He explained to me the type of cancer I had and what was to be the treatment I should have. He recommended that I start with chemotherapy (poison) to shrink the tumor and after that have an operation (cut) followed by radiation treatment (burn). I responded by quietly telling him that I wanted to try natural methods first. At first it seemed as if he had not heard me. But this time I did repeat what I had just said. I calmly spoke a little louder and told him again that I wanted to try natural methods first. He looked at me and just then seemed to realize I was a person, not just cancer patient # 500900903. Not only was I a person, I was also not going to accept the treatment he was offering me: I was not passively undergoing his recommended treatment. This realization did not do much for his bedside manner. His kindly demeanor dropped, his smile disappeared and, somewhat haughtily, he answered that he wasn't pleased and that he was against what I was going to do. He did not ask or try to find out why I was doing this, what I was planning to do, or who I was as a person.

I asked him exactly how long the chemo would take and he answered 3 months. I answered, "I would like to try natural methods for the same amount of time." I wanted to give myself 3 months to see if this could shrink the tumor. Again not asking me any questions, he repeated that he was not happy with this, and now spoke to me more in a way a parent speaks to a wayward child. How strange: it was not up to me to make this man happy or any other person for that matter. A calmness had overtaken me, and it was as if I were outside of myself watching me, asking this man intelligent eloquent questions. I was all those things, but I was also in a stressful situation that usually left me searching for words. Who was that person in the chair—was that really me?

I asked him what he felt the outcome of the chemotherapy would be. He answered that they were hoping for some shrinkage. I did not feel that undergoing such an invasive treatment in hopes that the tumor would shrink was good enough. Yes, the tumor could shrink but the damage to my body was a very high price to pay, and I told him this. He appeared to become defensive and started defending chemotherapy as I expected he would do. After all, this is what he believed in and so he needed to be able to defend his choices. His explanation was much the same as the answer the surgeon had given me: Chemotherapy is a systemic treatment, and it would travel throughout my entire body attacking and cleaning up possible stray cancer cells.

I responded that at this time we were not sure if there were any stray cancer cells, were we, because no test had been conducted to confirm or deny this. He felt that this was a dangerous thing for me to take a chance on because he knew how cancer cells behaved and, based on other people's cases and his knowledge of cancer, he wanted to take the secure route of attacking this cancer aggressively. Again, his answer made sense and sounded logical and previously, when I still held the belief that doctors were gods, I would not have questioned him, but I had begun to inform myself and from my reading I knew how destructive chemotherapy was to my already very weak immune system. Patients who have undergone chemotherapy have to be extremely careful with any type of attack on their body and even a simple flu virus could possibly be fatal. Months earlier, my niece had undergone chemotherapy for Leukemia and we all had to wear masks and gowns when we visited her in the hospital after her treatment because the risk of infections were so high. And if I were refusing chemotherapy on a whim, without substituting something else or not doing anything, that could be even more hazardous. But I was doing something; I was already actively supporting my immune system.

I asked him, "What if I had surgery combined with the other treatments I was currently undertaking?" I felt that if I had the surgery, I would have a fighting chance. His answer was again that this was not enough and that we needed to attack this disease using a systemic approach and this was chemotherapy before surgery to ensure we got the stray cancer cells.

I wanted to know what his answers would be about stimulating my immune system, so I asked him if instead of attacking my immune system even more there was not a known medical procedure that could help me stimulate and heal my immune system. He all but dismissed this question and tried to change the topic back to his knowledge and expertise around the three known methods used to combat cancer: chemotherapy (poison), radiation (burn) and surgery (cut). He did mention that there was an experimental study being done called stemcell treatment, but it was not yet available. He did not explain it to me.

When it became clear that I had made up my mind, the oncologist began to leave the room. But before he did, he had one parting shot left for me. Standing at the door, holding the door handle, he turned back to face me, looked sternly over his glasses and said;" well, I can't guarantee that we will save your breast." I was appalled, but again heard myself answer in the same calm manner, "I am more than just my breast, and I accept that responsibility."

The nurse also left, but before she did, she gave me information that at the cancer society's office that night there was a meeting for *Reach to Recovery*. The topic was boosting your immune system. She had heard me explain to the oncologist that this was what I was planning to do. Unknown to them (because they did not ask and I did not offer the information), I had already started my own battle plan and was following it by making a drastic change in my eating habits and by taking vitamin supplements the day I had read the articles Dr. Jones had given me. I felt, by boosting my own immune system, my body would stand a much better chance of fighting the cancer cells. The oncologist did not appear to put too much stock into that idea. His comments were that there were no documented cases to indicate that this had ever worked. I wonder if I am now a "documented case" or if they have decided that the reason I am alive is not due to alternative methods. After the nurse left the room, Jenni and I talked about that night's upcoming meeting. We decided to go to there together. We asked the nurse for the address and the meeting times.

After I got dressed, Jenni and I walked through the Oncology Department on our way to the stairs. It didn't take long before we became aware that where we walked all conversation between Medical Personnel stopped, and many of the nurses turned to look at us. Was I becoming paranoid or had they all been talking about me? Were they discussing the choice I made? It did appear that way.

That evening Jenni and I went to the meeting at the cancer society. We walked through the door, and this is what we saw: The room was already very full; it was buzzing with conversation; the women were mostly older (they looked to be in their late 50s); some were wearing turbans hiding their hairless heads, others wore obvious wigs; there was a small group of younger looking women sitting together; in the corner stood a table filled with coffee, black tea, and store bought cookies—no herbal tea, no juice, no fruit, no healthy snacks, not even fresh water. The only refreshments available were, according to the information I was reading to make myself informed, all things a woman with breast cancer should avoid eating or drinking. We both felt disappointed at the lack of nutritional information or nutritional support at a cancer support meeting and spoke of it briefly to each other. It was disappointing not to find anything healthy to snack on. Jenni and I decided not to eat or drink anything. We would drink water from the fountain in the hallway, or not have anything; even though I had already stopped drinking chlorinated tap water, because chlorine is a known cell killer. In the future I would be more prepared and bring a thermos filled with herbal tea wherever I went.

I felt eager anticipation. Would there be useful information for me that night? I was hoping there would be. I looked around the room and saw again that most women were much older than me. They all seemed to know each other; it felt like a social club. What a club to belong to—the breast cancer club (I do recognize that this was also a support group for women with breast cancer. And I feel that support groups play an important role in the recovery process). Most of the chairs were already taken, so after we put a nametag on, Jenni and I had to sit in the front row, center seats, not at all where I would normally have sat: I like sitting in the back, close to the exit so I can leave whenever I want if the meeting proved not to be worth my time. But that day we had no choice—if we wanted to hear the information or be able to have a seat, we had to take the front center seats.

The speaker, a young research doctor entered and was introduced. She was dressed stylishly in a short black dress. She had brought slides with her and started giving us a very intellectual scientific explanation of how far they had progressed in this field. I was questioning this in my mind. Had they really progressed far in the battle against cancer? It did not seem far at all. It was only from a medical/scientific perspective. She talked about removing healthy cells from the woman's body, taking them to the lab and "treating" them. After the treatment they would re-insert these treated cells back into the body of a person with cancer. She was explaining the treatment the oncologist had mentioned earlier that day: stem cell treatment. She explained that it was still in the exploratory stage. I did not listen too closely but to me it sounded like it was about finding a cure inside a lab—away from the person, treating the cancer cells as something separate from the person whose body they were living in. It was about dissecting a whole and then reassembling it, not looking at the whole and trying to find a cure from within. It seemed backwards to me, and it did not agree with my emerging views.

I realized that I had accepted and adopted the views of the doctors whose articles I had read a short time earlier. Since that first Monday, after I had seen Dr. Jones and had received the articles from him I had been gathering more information and found that chemotherapy was based on mustard gas which had further shocked me. I had also realized the incredible effect our diets have on our health, and that if we do not put proper fuel, for lack of a better word, in our bodies we can become very ill.

This was exactly what had happened to me. I also had begun to inform myself more on the mind/body connection and how our emotions and feelings influence our health, as well. I had not yet begun to address this aspect of my illness, but I was becoming aware that this too had possibly contributed to my depressed immune system. As much as a hug and feeling good elevates our immune system, the reverse is also true for stress and unhappiness: they can produce a strain on how our bodies fight illnesses.

My views were becoming clearer and more pronounced, and they included the whole picture, not only the person, but their lives and lifestyles as well. I did not adhere to the Descartian belief that illness is something to be taken out of the person and treated away from them. My beliefs were directly opposed to that and much closer to the Asian and Native American beliefs that the illness is the symptom and is a part of a much larger whole and that it is not to be looked at separately away from the person. Because if that is done, then yes, the illness can be treated and possibly even cured, but it remains a band-aid solution if the underlying cause is not addressed. I felt that most practitioners in the mainstream medical community were not yet open to looking at illnesses that way. I was glad that my family doctor was more open minded and extremely grateful for the support from Dr. Jones.

During my last visit with my family doctor she had told me about a lecture she had attended by a prominent local oncologist. He had told them about three women getting identical cancer. They were all the same age and their treatments would also have been identical. Yet one woman's cancer would go into remission and later return, another would die within months, and the third would completely recover. He had told his audience, "we are missing something; we are not considering the host!" Contemplating what my doctor had told me, it was clear to me that the speaker I was presently listening to did not appear to be interested in the host, either—her interest was only in the cancer cells to be treated and cured in a lab, separate from "the host."

What I had wanted to hear and why I had come, was to find out how I could stimulate my immune system and increase my healthy cells while keeping them in my body. Were there foods I could eat which supported, others which should be eliminated? After all, my body, me, had created this tumor; was it also then not possible for my body, me, to destroy this tumor if I gave myself, my body, the tools to do so? I was repeating to myself what I had learned so far about cancer. Fact: our bodies create cancer cells daily, but in a healthy body they are destroyed by our own immune system; fact: cancer cells are the weaker cells, so they can more easily be destroyed. That is how cancer was explained according to the books and articles I was reading. But that was not what this speaker with her scientific mind seemed to be telling us. This was supposed to be a talk on strengthening your immune system. When would she talk to us about that?

Her lecture part of the evening was now over. She had not given us any information about naturally boosting our immune system. She had only explained this new scientific technique called stem cell treatment. She opened up the floor for discussion and questions. Many of the questions from the older women were about a cure for "our daughters." I thought, "What about a cure for us? I want to live; I don't want a cure later, for the next generation: I want a cure now, for me!"

I was sitting there pondering these thoughts when I was suddenly catapulted back into the room. A woman sitting next to the wall on the left side of the room was asking a question about using alternative methods. Hearing those words had brought my awareness back into the room. The young doctor began to answer the question, but instead of looking at the person who had asked the question, and who was not sitting anywhere near me, she appeared to be looking directly at me! I wanted to look over my shoulder to see if maybe she was directing her answer at someone behind me, but I didn't because she was looking directly into my eyes. She spoke, very seriously, and her words appeared to be specifically directed at me. She said very insistently, while looking into my eyes, "Alternative methods are very dangerous and should not be used instead of conventional treatments!"

I felt as if I had entered the twilight zone. Was she really speaking directly at me? Did she know who I was, that I had been at the cancer clinic earlier that day to see the oncologist, and that I had told him that I was refusing conventional treatment and would instead focus on what the mainstream medical community called "alternative methods"? If so, how did she know me? I had never seen her before. Had she really directed her answer at me, or was I now becoming seriously paranoid? No, I was not imagining it, she really did speak directly to me, and Jenni confirmed it later in the car. Jenni had also heard and seen the person by the wall ask the question about alternative methods. And she, too, had seen and heard how this young doctor had then turned to me and by looking directly at me had answered the question asked by someone who was not even remotely sitting near me. But if this were true how did she know who I was, that I was the woman choosing alternative methods? Then it suddenly occurred to me how she knew who I was: I was wearing a nametag! And because I was sitting in the front row she could read my name. Had she been told by the nurse or the oncologist that I would be there and what my name was and to look out for me? Was it her aim to dissuade me from using the road I had chosen? I don't know the answer to that.

Jenni and I left immediately after the lecture was over. We discussed our experience and our impressions of the "The breast cancer Club" during our drive home. I knew that this was not a place where I would go to find comfort, support, or information. It appeared that most of the women present had seemed far too resigned about their fate; they all appeared to implicitly trust their doctors. It also appeared that they submissively followed the advice given by their doctors. I did not want to take such a passive role. I was beginning to feel quite alone. I wanted to find another person who was traveling the same road I was on and who was making similar choices to the ones I had. Would I find such a person, or would I have to travel this journey alone? I had people I could talk to, they supported my choices, but they did not have cancer. Would they make the same decisions I had made if they had? It is often easy to say you will take a certain course of action when you are not directly in that situation. However, when it concerns you personally, you may make a different choice. I wanted someone to talk to who was facing the same illness and who was making similar choices to the one I was making.

Chapter Nine

Listening to My Inner Voice...

The next day started like any other day. For me, it was the day that I had to tell my family and friends that I was, at this point, choosing not to have conventional cancer treatment and would focus on using a more natural holistic approach, instead. As I had expected, this information was met with mixed reviews. Some people did not know what to say to me, only to say, as I found out, plenty behind my back. Most of that somehow made its way back to me anyway by other "well meaning" people who felt I should hear this. Others would tell me to my face that they disagreed with my choice and tried to make me change my mind. I acknowledge that most were confronting their own fears about this frightening disease.

But as much as most people were opposed to my course of action, there were a very small number of people who unconditionally supported my choice. My supporters were Jenni, my friend; Dan, my boss; Stephen Jones, my Chiropractor; and my friend Ieke in Holland. It was a very small group. The people I had previously counted as my closest friends by and large did not support my choice. Having to continuously defend my chosen road to many of my friends and family left me feeling dejected and forlorn. I decided not to spend more energy explaining my choices. I needed all my energy to focus on healing and to strengthen my immune system. I did not have the luxury to spend energy to keep having to defend my choice to people who did not seem to understand or would not understand. But I was actively looking for more support.

I had heard that there was a woman connected with the hospital who lead a yoga group for people facing cancer. I was feeling hopeful that there I would find someone who also had breast cancer and who was traveling on the same road I was. I phoned her—but she never called me back! Also, *Reach to Recovery* usually contacts women newly diagnosed with breast cancer within days of their diagnosis. I did not receive a phone call or any other form of contact from them, either. When my sister Anneke, asked the cancer clinic in July why I was not receiving any support, her question was not directly answered. However, a letter sent to my doctor by the cancer clinic, mentioned that support had been offered to me, and that I had refused it.

This is not true. I was choosing not to submit myself to conventional cancer treatment at this time, but I was not refusing support. By now I realized how important support was, and I was actively trying to find more of it. I had phoned Ieke in Holland who immediately started sending me information from Holland about alternative methods. She also sent me encouraging letters and cards. Her friendship became an important lifeline. The books and articles she sent me were very interesting. I realized that in Holland it was much easier for people to choose alternative methods because their health care paid for many so called alternative treatments. One book especially that Ieke had sent me on diet and nutrition called *Moerman's Diet* supported my "new" eating habits.

Many of the people who did not agree with my choice would, once they had processed this, return and try to encourage as best as they could. But it always felt tentative, the way one supports a child's "foolish" choice, "Knowing" as adults there is a "better" way, the adult's way. But it was still support, and I needed all I could get in whatever form it came, so I eagerly accepted their support and felt surrounded by their love.

Meanwhile, my strongest ally was Jenni. Together, we toured local farmers' markets. We ate raw organic food, or steamed our food to keep it very close to its original source, so that it preserved as many nutrients as possible, thus giving my body potent fuel. We went on many walks and had long talks. On Jenni's recommendation, because she had spoken to him about me, I went to see the minister of her church. He asked if he could be part of my team. At that time, I had not realized I had a team, but when he asked if he could join my team, I realized that I did, indeed, have a team of supporters. It was a group of people surrounding me who encouraged me, who cheered me on and gave me information. I had to fight alone, go on an uncharted road which lay before me, but many people were there to lend support. Not only my core supporters who cheered me unconditionally—Stephen, Dan, Ieke and Jenni— but a larger group of many other people as well. People who backed me in the best way they could.

So when Duncan, the minister, asked to be part of my team, it made me realize that I did have a team of supporters. The backing consisted of many forms of support. It included a wall of prayer around me. Prayers were said for me around the world, not only in Canada and Holland, where family and friends prayed, but in many other countries as well. People I didn't know, but who were known to the women I worked with, all prayed, too. During 1996, I was working as a Day Home Supervisor and many of the women who ran Day Homes came from different parts of the world. They had come from Afghanistan, Iran, Shri-Lanka, Greece, Denmark, the Philippines, and Vietnam. They all asked what they could do. I asked them to pray for me and, if they did not pray, to send me white light. I knew and felt that these prayers had formed a wall of prayer around me. There are many documented miracles in spiritual circles attributed to people being prayed over.

The next seven weeks seemed much longer than they actually were. My awareness of life was enormously heightened. Everything appeared larger than life (strange choice of words, since I was fighting for my life). I was also fine-tuning my battle plan. Not everything I did was positive or worked for me. I went to see a local herbalist who sold me several remedies. They made me violently ill, so I stopped them immediately. I also saw a Russian doctor in a health food store who told me that my relationship with food had to change. I felt she was right about that. However she could not offer me anything else worthwhile. I continued my search and my research. People were trying to be helpful and sent me articles about "alternative" methods.

During this time, something unusual was happening in my house. Many things, too many for me to miss, but so that I had to take notice, were breaking down. One after the other, appliances broke or broke down as if in sympathy with what was happening inside my body. It was as if to mirror to me that inside my body, cells were breaking down to form the mutant malignant cancer cells. First my dishwasher broke, after that the lawnmower, followed by the vacuum cleaner. Also, countless light bulbs burned out, one after the other. Then the television broke down and, simultaneously, both bathroom fans stopped working. On and on it went: Next, the toaster became toast and the fan belt in the car broke and a cement block on the front lawn cracked. It was the strangest thing; it just kept going, one thing after another kept breaking down or breaking in my surroundings. I had never, previously, and have never since, had so many things break down in my house so close together in time as they did that summer in 1996.

During the fight, I would lose a special friend. She, who had played an extremely important role, both as friend and to encourage me during my pregnancy and the raising of Vincent, was mostly absent in this. I'm still not sure why this happened. Was it too difficult for her, a traditional nurse, to support my choice for alternative medicine? I don't know. What I do know is that whenever she came for a visit, she only talked about her own life. There appeared to be no room for me to talk to her about what was happening to me. It was as if she did not want to hear it or talk about it. Was this how her fear manifested itself? Again, I don't know. She also appeared not to understand my changed eating and living habits. Many people did not, but they kept their comments to themselves. She did not keep her comments to herself and would often make, what felt like, sarcastic comments.

When I tried to explain that I did not want to eat anything that included preservatives her response was that she needed all the preservatives she could get so she could be preserved.

However, when I stopped drinking coffee and eating high fat and unhealthy food, it was as if she took this as a personal attack. My loneliest time with her came when Vincent and I met her and her children at Callaway Park, a local amusement park. She had offered to bring food for all of us to eat. When she opened the cooler it was obvious that there was nothing to eat for me in the picnic lunch. She was well aware of my changed eating habits. The container she had brought was filled with food, but in it there was only white bread spread with butter layered with processed meat and cheese whiz, and she had brought only donuts and cookies for desert. The choices of drinks were coffee or carbonated soft drinks. I felt very hurt, and I didn't know what to say. To make matters even worse, she made a comment to Vincent that he could still come to her house whenever he wanted fat or sugar. This seemed to say clearly that she did know that I had eliminated both from my diet. When I heard her say that, I felt even more upset and close to tears. This was a woman I had long considered to be one of my best friends. Vincent looked at me and I could see in his face that he was aware of how hurtful her comment was to me. He would later tell me that he knew how much her words hurt me, but being only 14, he had not known what to say in my defense. His eyes had supported me but, as he said, he had wanted to give me more support, but did not know how.

I believe that at that point our friendship was given a mortal blow, from which it has not recovered to this day. I wonder if she knew what happened to me that day and how alone I felt in her company during a time when I needed her support not her criticism. I miss the friend who fell away but in the summer of '96 I did not have the energy to try and build a bridge or repair the damaged friendship. I was using all the energy I had for the fight of my life. She did not try to reach out to me in any way I recognized, and today a rift continues to exist between us that time has not helped heal.

Another friend's fears and concerns manifested itself in a different way. Happily, this friendship survived, but it happened only after I had taken some distance. I had explained to this friend about my choice not to follow the oncologist's recommendations and the changes I had made in my diet and lifestyle. She told me in response that I was in shock and should go back to the cancer clinic and start the treatment immediately. I tried to explain to her why I had made the choice I had, but she would not or could not hear me. Every time we met or talked on the phone she continued to try and convince me that I only had one choice—that was to use mainstream medicine. I tried a few more times to explain my choice to her, but I could not make myself understood. I could feel myself using energy during these conversations, energy I desperately needed for myself. It was clear that I needed all I had to continuously defend myself against a deadly enemy. I would not spend it trying to convince people what I was doing and why. It was with this realization that I told her that if she could not support me and that if I had to defend myself every time we spoke, I could not have contact with her, not until she could become more supportive of my choice. I do believe that what she said came from her heart and that she was very afraid for my well being.

During our separation, she continued to try behind the scenes to "help" dissuade me from what she saw as a foolish choice. She phoned Duncan the minister to ask him to please try and talk some sense into me. He did give me the message and told me that my friend had called him and what she had said. But he supported my choice. He and his wife were great believers in the benefits of juicing and eating healthy. He gave me a juicer, and I incorporated drinking fresh juices into my treatment regimen as well.

My friend's comments, however, had not fallen on deaf ears. I looked deep into myself: Perhaps she was right—could I be in shock? Was I in denial, as she claimed? And if I were, would I be able to see it myself? I had to know, so I asked Dr. Jones, before I had one of my *Microcurrent Electrical Stimulation* sessions, if he felt that I was in shock or denial. His reply was that he felt

ROW, ROW, ROW MY BOAT

that I was neither in shock nor in denial. In his opinion, I was quite aware of what cancer is. I knew that I had felt both shock and denial earlier, after hearing the initial diagnosis from my family doctor. Dr. Jones validated my budding trust in myself; I knew deep inside me that he was right, but I felt not yet strong enough in this knowledge to fully trust my own inner knowing; yet, it did help to hear him say the words and how he perceived the situation; it helped strengthen my increasing reliance in my own feelings.

During this time, I also asked Dr. Jones pointedly on several occasions what he would do if he were in my shoes. He would not give me an answer. He did not give me an answer because it would have influenced me. He left it to me to decide. He provided me with support and information, yet at no point did he tell me what to do.

On a few occasions I became very angry and upset with him for not giving me direct advice, yet even then he would not tell me what to do. He knew I was very angry with him, but he remained in integrity and did not waver by telling me what I should or should not do. At a time when so many people felt that they had the right to tell me what actions to take, this man supported me in my choice whatever that was, but left me to decide for myself what road I would take. What I received from him was a great gift. He did not make the choice for me; instead, he allowed me to listen to my own inner knowing, so that I could decide for myself what to do, based on what was right for me.

Chapter Ten

Psychosynthesis

More was needed, I needed something else....
With all the vitamin supplements I was taking, the immune stimulating treatments from Dr. Jones, plus the change in diet, and the wall of prayer around me, I still had a nagging feeling that I needed to do something else. The little voice I was now beginning to listen to more intently was whispering that even by doing all of this, more was needed. But the question was what? And where would I find it? A friend's name kept "popping" into my mind. I knew she was closely connected to the alternative healing community in Calgary. So I phoned her and I told her what I was facing, and I how I "felt" that she had some information I needed.

She thought that she knew what it was and she gave me the name of a man who works with crystals. She explained to me that he has worked in hospitals with cancer patients using his crystals. We made plans to visit and she would look up his name and phone number. A few days later I met with her and at that time she not only presented me with his business card, but also gave me a newspaper article about what this man does. I took them home with me and I promptly lost both. She phoned me a few days later to find out if I had been able to connect with this man; when I told her I had lost his phone number, she gave it to me once more. The same thing happened again: I lost the number before I could use it.

After I had lost it twice I realized that this was not the person I needed. But I did continue to feel that my friend knew someone I had to meet. So I phoned her again and told her that I felt that the man with the crystals was not the person I should see, but that there was someone else she knew. She did not know immediately who it could be, but she answered that she would reflect on it. Not long after that, she called me back and she sounded very excited. She told me that a name had come to her mind and she questioned why she had not thought about her before. She explained that she *knew* who it was I had to see and she told me the person's name.

She said, "It is Julie Alexander!" As soon as she said Julie's name I immediately "knew" that she was the person I had to meet with. I did not have a clue what she did or who she was, but somehow I "knew" she was the one. While my friend and I were talking on the phone, she received a signal on her phone that someone else was calling. She excused herself for a minute to check who it was and promised to return immediately to our call. When she came back on the line she told me, somewhat awed, "You'll never guess who was on the other line?" But I knew and I was not at all surprised when she told me that it had been Julie on the other line. They had not spoken to each other for a few months; yet, during our phone conversation, while she was telling me about Julie, Julie herself had called. I felt this was a sign and a validation that I should go and meet with Julie.

After I was given Julie's phone number I called her as soon as I got off the phone. I didn't have to explain who I was because my friend had given Julie the short version when she had spoken with her earlier. She agreed to see me that afternoon. That same afternoon, I was also to meet my Dutch friend Ieke. Ieke was in Canada with her family for a vacation, but everyone else was sight-seeing which left us free to spend a few hours together, just the two of us. I would meet with Julie first and then visit with Ieke.

I drove to Julie's house where she greeted me with a warm friendly smile. She explained that she is a Psychosynthesis guide. I had never heard of Psychosynthesis and did not know anything about it. She invited me in. The room she preceded me into was decorated beautifully and eclectically. It was decorated with plants, art, and antiques; it felt soothing and serene.

The first thing Julie told me was to slow down. I was very surprised because I thought I was calm and had slowed down. In any case, if I was not exactly calm on the inside, I did feel that surely I presented a calm exterior. But Julie saw through my exterior and knew intuitively that I was anything but calm. Julie asked me if I wanted to do a guided visualization. I nodded, and she asked me to close my eyes and, in a calm voice, she told me to relax. When I was in a relaxed state, she asked me to "see" the speed. I tried, but all I could "see" was a blur and I told her so. With my eyes still closed it was as if I were "seeing" something move across my vision with such speed that I could not see what it was.

I told her I couldn't recognize what it was because it was going too fast. She asked me to freeze frame the speed: I did so, and at that time, I could see that it was a train. She asked me where it was going. I told her nowhere and knew that to be true. She then asked me to open my eyes; when I did, we discussed how I had internalized speed into my life and into my body. It was true: I was always rushing off to something, to somewhere: so many things happening in my life, so much to occupy my time with. I had been very busy with all my jobs before the cancer hit; I had made some changes but *I* had not really changed. I had merely exchanged one form of busy-ness with another. I was now very busy with learning about cancer and being focused on fighting it. Busy, busy, busy....

I felt I had slowed down because I was no longer working at all my jobs. The reality was that I had only stopped working at two part-time jobs but still had the other two as well as my full time job. I certainly had not slowed down sufficiently. In me there was still speed, much like a train on a very fast track. It is very difficult for a train to slow down, because there is so much weight behind it, and it is even more difficult to change course. I had made numerous external changes, and I was trying to change the direction that my life had taken. But I needed to go inside to get to the controls. Psychosynthesis would help me do this.

July explained that it was very important that I slow down. But somehow to me being busy meant that I was alive, and I told Julie this. She asked me if I felt a tree was alive.

I said, "Yes, a tree is alive."

"Is it moving?"

I shook my head.

"Is it rushing anywhere?"

Again I shook my head, I began to understand what she meant and she clarified it even more.

"A tree is very much alive and yet very grounded at the same time," she explained.

I nodded in reluctant agreement. What she was saying was certainly true: I had to admit that to myself, but I was still very much caught up in my own belief that to be really alive meant speed and moving from one place to another.

She continued, "For you and for anyone else who has internalized the speed from our busy world it is very important to slow down and become grounded again. There is a very simple thing you can do to help yourself with that. Find a tree, the larger the better, and hug it or sit against it. Try to feel its aliveness and its groundedness." I could feel that this was a very important thing for me to do.

Then Julie explained to me what Psychosynthesis is. It is a life long process to help us understand ourselves better. I was to find out that it would require a great deal, and that the resistance I had encountered from friends and family was nothing compared to the resistance I would encounter in myself.

Psychosynthesis in its simplest form is a name for the process of growth. It is based on the belief that life has caused separation within us and that, through a guided process, we can bring these separate parts of ourselves back into unity and bring about synthesis

She explained that through Psychosynthesis we can learn to consciously choose to support that process.

What was really important for me to hear was when Julie said that unlike most forms of psychotherapy, Psychosynthesis recognizes a part of us that is difficult to name. This part is referred to as "higher" or "deeper". She said that, in any case, it is for us the source of inspiration, guidance, comfort, strength, peace, hope. Psychosynthesis calls this part the "self" and she explained that integration, synthesis, or unification of the personality, happens around this "self."

Julie continued by telling me that the "self" has two aspects - the personal and the transpersonal, and that synthesis happens in two stage: first the personal, followed by the transpersonal. I wasn't entirely sure what she meant with transpersonal, but I understood the part about the "self." I was already beginning more and more to listen to and be guided by this part of me, my higher self. I wanted to learn more about it and discover ways to access my higher self more.

Julie continued by saying that one of the strengths of Psychosynthesis is that it provides practical methods to recognize and access the "higher" or "deeper" part of ourselves, so that the process of growth happens according to an "inner wisdom." She said that this means that in accessing this truly empowering part of ourselves, our own inner self is not violated or imposed upon: It is allowed to unfold at its own speed, and according to its own pattern. It was good for me to hear that Psychosynthesis honors all parts of our being, teaching us to work through blocks that hinder growth, without creating further blocks in the process.

The more Julie explained, the more I liked what she told me about Psychosynthesis, especially that its goal is integration and wholeness. She explained that the therapy would have aspects of one-on-one meetings with her, but that group meetings were also a very important part of what Psychosynthesis is. She had a group thatch had just started and if I wanted to I could join it. Julie then told me that in Psychosynthesis some of the techniques she uses are guided imagery, self-identification, meditation, development of the will, symbolic art work, journal keeping, and development of intuition. She said that the emphasis is on encouraging an ongoing process of growth that can bring about a more joyful, balanced actualization of one's life.

Julie continued as she said, "As this process goes forward, you gain the freedom of choice." All of this sounded like something which I very much wanted for my life. Whether it was my higher self or another part of me "speaking" I don't know but I could "feel" that Psychosynthesis would be of incredible benefit to me in my fight against cancer. The more Julie explained about this process, the stronger the feeling became that this was what had been the missing component and that in addition to the other aspects of my "fight plan" my "action plan" this needed to be added. I was fighting on a physical level: change of diet, supplements; M.E.S. (Dr. Jones); spiritual level: prayer; intellectual level: research and becoming informed; and now, with Psychosynthesis, I could add the emotional component. Not only would it benefit the emotional aspect but also add to the spiritual and intellectual side as well.

Julie gave me two more piece of information before I left, but I was already convinced that this was to be part of my plan; hearing what she had to say confirmed that I must add the emotional component. She said that one major difficulty is learning to act "from center" and not to react from false *identifications*. She explained what this meant and said that we may (falsely) identify, for example with a temporary feeling such as fear or anger, and lose or distort our true perspective. Or we may become identified with one of our "sub personalities"— those semi-autonomous and often contradictory aspects of ourselves that follow a predictable, pre-programmed routine when evoked by a certain set of circumstances. She explained that this was the difference between reacting from an almost automatic emotional base to responding from an awakened place. Once more, I only understood some of what she was saying but based on that level of understanding, I told her that I definitely wanted to learn all these things and that I felt it would help me tremendously in the battle I was fighting.

Julie then continued by explaining that in Psychosynthesis much of the basic work is aimed at recognizing and harmonizing sub personalities, so that we are no longer helplessly controlled by them. Doing this involves learning the central process of "disidentification" from all that is not the "self", and "self-identification" or the realization of our true identity as a center of awareness and will. Through this development, we free ourselves from helpless reaction to unwanted inner impulses, and to the expectations of others. We become truly "centered" and gradually become able to follow a path in accordance with what is best within each of us.

Again, there was so much information, so many new ideas and thoughts for me to process. I had only grasped portions of it, because so much of what Julie said I had never heard explained like that before, but I "knew" enough of the ideas to convince me that this was what I wanted to learn. I understood about automatic emotional reactions to different situations. Ten years earlier, Vincent had been hurt playing behind my parents' car while visiting them. He had large scrapes on his legs and it was quite painful for him, but other than that he was unhurt. However, when Pa later that day told me about his accident, my reaction had been so strong that it had taken me by surprise.

It was too strong for the situation; after I had calmed down, I had tried to analyze what had happened. It was then that I remembered that when I was four years old I had witnessed a little girl being hit by a car. My parents did not know I had been there because I had not told anyone. It had happened in front of my school while I was waiting outside for my chaperone. I had internalized this event, so when more than 25 years later my own little four year old child had an accident that involved a car I had spontaneously regressed back into my own four year old self. And that was the part that had reacted so strongly. So when Julie explained about "automatic" responses from a younger self I knew exactly what she meant because I had experienced just that myself ten years earlier. I had never done anything with this information, but now I was offered a chance to learn how not to react and respond instead.

Before I left, Julie recommended that I should go and find a tree, hug it, and sit under it and allow it to help me slow down.

After I left Julie, I drove to Heritage Park where I was to meet Ieke. While waiting for my friend, I found a tree and sat under it, leaning against it. I was trying to feel the steady slow pulse of life in the tree. I could imagine it, but I could not really feel it; but even so, I was beginning to feel calmer after my session with Julie and from sitting next to a tree. When Ieke walked through the gate, she saw me sitting under the tree, and I explained to her why I had chosen to wait for her there. Our hello hug was grave compared to the jubilant hello hug we had shared earlier that year when she had visited before I had received the cancer diagnosis. So much had changed since we had last seen each other not much earlier in the year. Then we had not seen each other in years; yet, the years were bridged effortlessly. What had taken place in the weeks since I had last seen her, however, was not so easily bridged.

We spent the afternoon in my small backyard. My garden that day was simply a square patch of grass left by the previous owners. Next to the house there were decorative stones to cover the earth. There were no flower beds. But I wanted to change that. I had already decided that I wanted to fill my little back yard with flowers and shrubs. I had also made up my mind that I would not plant any annual bedding plants, instead I had decided that I only wanted to plant perennial plants in my little backyard. I felt that if I put annual plants in my garden it would show that I did not have enough faith that I would see next year. I was going to plant only perennial plants, and I was going to be there to watch them grow, year after year.

Planting annuals flowers to me meant defeat. Annuals do not survive the winter, and I wanted to make sure that I did, and I wanted whatever I chose to grow in my garden, that summer, to be there to welcome me in the spring of the following year. I was not going to die, and I did not want anything else around me to die either, including the plants in my garden.

I not only intended to be there for the next year, I had now decided that I would live to be a 100 something. I had changed the number from the initial response I had earlier given my family doctor. Instead of living to be 90 years, I was going to live to be 100 something years.

In the summer of 1996, my little garden flourished and grew very lovely, but something else was growing as well. The tumor continued to grow, ever larger and larger. During the day I would often touch it to check its size and it seemed that the more afraid I felt, the bigger the tumor grew. It looked as if it was fed by my fear, and it was almost as if I could see it grow. Whenever I touched the tumor and felt its growing size, the icy fingers of fear would clutch my heart and fill me with immeasurable alarm....

Chapter Eleven

Feeling backed into a corner

THE LOSS OF EMPOWERMENT AND COURAGE; JULY '96

My sister Anneke, who lived in Ottawa, had come for a visit with her family. She is the sister I have the closest connection with. She wanted to know how I was doing, and we discussed my growing tumor. I had not officially measured it, but by touching it with my fingers, I could feel that it was getting larger and that the hardness in my breast, which I could trace with my fingers, was now about the size of a tennis ball. During the many long conversations I had with Anneke, I explained to her that I felt that if the tumor were cut out of my breast, I would have a chance to fight the disease. I also gave her an account of my earlier visit with the surgeon and how, even then, I had felt that if I could just have the surgery, I would have a fighting chance. But the only surgeon I knew had sent me to the oncologist while explaining to me I needed to have chemotherapy first. We discussed the possibility that I should go back to this surgeon and ask her to perform surgery: it was the best idea we could come up with. Something needed to be done, because the tumor continued growing. We decided to go and see the surgeon together. She would be my support while I would try to convince the surgeon I wanted the operation.

The next day, I phoned the hospital to try and get the earliest possible appointment. I was very surprised when I was told that I could come in early the next day. When we arrived for my appointment, we were taken into a small little room and again did not have to wait very long, at all. Initially, the surgeon was calm; however, when she became aware of my request for surgery and that I was still refusing chemotherapy, she became increasingly agitated and appeared to be very angry. At one point, she pointed her finger at me and declared sharply, "YOU ARE DICTATING YOUR OWN TREATMENT!"

Being spoken to in this manner was shocking but, somehow, I remained composed and answered her calmly, "I thought I had a choice." Her reply was again very intense when she almost shouted, "YOU DON'T HAVE A CHOICE!"

I didn't want to fight or argue with her because I was there with a purpose: I wanted her to do my surgery. My appointment with her was to request that she surgically remove the tumor. So I explained again to her that I felt that if the tumor was cut out, I would have a fighting chance to beat this disease. Again, she disagreed and flatly refused to perform surgery on my breast unless I had chemotherapy first. She felt that it would be a waste of time if I had surgery without chemotherapy. And I was saying "No" refusing to have chemotherapy. She told me the same things again I had earlier been told by the oncologist. It was like having the same conversation all over again: Yes, I realized the logic in what they were saying; yes, I understood their reasoning that Chemotherapy was a systemic approach and that it had a greater chance of finding and destroying stray cells than surgery. But I also knew that Chemotherapy destroys immune systems and would destroy mine. Not only would the stray cells be destroyed, but my immune system as well. It was a very high price to pay for finding and destroying stray cancer cells.

But what about the risk I was taking by not finding and destroying the stray cells: Would I pay with my life? Would I have enough time with the holistic methods I was using to turn this horrible disease around—not just turn it around, but stop it in its tracks, then try and reverse the damage it was doing in my body? I desperately wanted answers and tried to find them as quickly as I could, knowing full well time was crucial and that I did not have much time to dilly dally or give myself a false assurance that all would be well. What was I to do? I know that this surgeon gave me the only information she could, based on her education, training, and current knowledge. As far as she was concerned, I did have only one choice, and I recognize that her words were based on what she knew and that from this stand point she was trying to give me the best advise she knew and that was to follow the path she and the oncologist had decided on.

And so she gave me all her reasoning from her vantage point, and I gave her mine. We were locked in a horrible impasse: one that neither one of us would win. I was standing firm by my convictions, and she was by hers. It felt like we were going around in circles, and when it became clear that the surgeon would not budge from her position, Anneke and I left. I was feeling very dejected; I also felt as if I had been in a boxing ring. I could feel the effects of this altercation in my body: A deep weariness had settled like a cape on my shoulders. I felt as if I had just fought 10 rounds boxing. Any time I encountered anyone in the mainstream medical field where there was only room for what they felt was the "best" method to use, I felt fearful, anxious, and powerless.

After the visit with the surgeon, Anneke and I went to the cancer library and signed out books on breast cancer. I was not at any time uninformed—I read and read and read all I could about this disease and became ever more informed. What I did learn was that even though the names of the treatment may have changed, the methods had not: It was still Cut (surgery), Poison (chemotherapy), and Burn (radiation).

Meanwhile I was struggling financially. I had barely been able to survive on 1 full-time and 4 part-time jobs, before I became sick. Supporting Vincent and myself now was becoming nearly impossible. The cost of the vitamins and shark cartilage alone was astronomical. I was only able to pay portions of my utility bills. There was also the increased cost of eating healthy. Strangely enough, in our very rich Western world, it is much cheaper to eat unhealthy fatty and over-processed foods, than it is to eat whole, organic healthy foods. The financial burden increased my already very high stress level.

I was also paying for my Psychosynthesis sessions with Julie. Julie's fees were reasonable, and she was doing everything to help by allowing me to pay in installments spread over a generous time period. But my financial load was so strained that even having to pay a few dollars broke the bank. I had heard that the cancer clinic employed a social worker; perhaps she could tell me where I could get some financial help. It was help I desperately needed to stay afloat.

I was not only battling a life-threatening disease—I was now battling poverty, as well. So much stress—my energy was beginning to wane, and I was getting scared. The tumor in my breast now felt huge—it felt like an orange, and I could feel that another lump had begun to form in my arm pit; it was the same size as the original lump had been when I first found it at the end of April. It was now July. The fight was getting harder and harder—could I keep it up; would I be able to turn the tide in time, before it got me?

I booked a visit with the Social Worker. She, too, must have heard about my choice of treatment because from the moment I met her, she appeared very antagonistic towards me. She began to ask me questions, supposedly to assess my needs, but it felt more like I was being cross examined. At one point she even asked me if I were suicidal. I answered her, somewhat surprised, that "NO," I was not. Then she continued, very sternly, by reminding me that I had to think of my son. I replied that I always thought of him, but that this time I also thought of myself, and I had to do this for me. She seemed very angry and upset with me. During the first half of my meeting with her, I did not know what to do. I felt bewildered much, like a student called into the principal's office to be called to task. But it didn't last long because I was beginning to have a stronger voice and to speak up for myself. I realized I did not have to sit there and be treated like a delinquent child.

I wanted to get out of this person's office, but before I did,

I spoke out. I told her how I felt and that I had come to her seeking support, but that I was not feeling that she was helping me at all. I was surprised when she agreed with me that it was true that she could not help me. She also made it very clear that there was no financial aid available for me. I had heard from other people that they did receive financial help but, perhaps based on my choices, I did not qualify. She did not ask me what my income was or what my financial needs were. She just told me point blanc that there was no financial aid available for me. I was a single mom on a very limited income: If financial aid is available, I am very curious about who qualifies. To her credit, she did tell me where I could park for free in the residential area, blocks away from the hospital. It was a small success, but it helped. It meant I had to walk for 10 -15 minutes, but saving the money for parking did help.

There were also no parking passes available for my use in the hospital parking lot, no other means of support that she could offer me. Again, later, I was to find out that other people were offered free parking passes for use in the parking lot next to the hospital. But they were not there for me. I told her there was no point for us to continue and that I was leaving: Another round of boxing, feeling more exhausted after I left than before I went in.

I needed support and she was not able to give it. She had made it very clear to me that she did not support my choice of treatment. The message I received from this was that only people who choose the "right" treatment receive other support. In these people's mind, I only had one choice and that was to do it their way.

But the tumor kept growing, and growing. I kept trying to do all I could, drinking freshly made juice daily, avoiding fat in my diet, and drinking Essiac Tea. Further, I had added Taheebo tea, which was another healing tea; I was taking all my supplements; eating organic, unprocessed fresh foods, including 15 grain breads and brown rice.

I was going to Julie for Psychosynthesis, and I was discovering more and more about myself. Psychosynthesis was helping me to identify personality parts that are in control at any given time and how they are responsible for how we react to a number of situations. I was discovering that a part of me wanted to die. This was a very important discovery, especially because I was dealing with a potentially deadly disease and was far closer to death than normal.

With the help of Julie, I dialogued with that part of me and discovered that a little three-year-old part of me felt very lost in this world and wanted to die. This three-year-old self had been trying to kill herself for a very long time. As I became more in touch with that part, I remembered that at that age I had been to the beach with an aunt and uncle, and I had been walking into the water. I had wanted to keep walking, but a stranger had seen me and had turned me around. I remembered crying profusely because of the frustration of not having been successful at ending my life at age three.

Psychosynthesis was providing me with tools and techniques so that when I discovered such a part I could ask it questions. I was also learning it was possible to have conflicting parts and that when this is so it is important to facilitate an agreement between all so that instead of spinning your wheels with inner conflict, you are able to go on with life.

I was discovering another part and this one was a very angry part, which was holding on to a very old anger. I had read that many people believe that a tumor sometimes represents anger, so was it possible that by repressing this anger, I had started growing a tumor? As I continued learning this, I realized I was on a journey of self-discovery into myself. Often, it was very painful; yet, when release came, lightness came over me and enabled me to continue on this journey.

I was seeing Dr. Jones several times a week for the M. E. S. treatments. People continued praying and because of this, I was still surrounded by a wall of prayer. Ieke continued sending me encouragement through phone calls, letters, and cards.

Even with all of this, I was beginning to feel like I was sinking into quicksand. I was beginning to waver in my choice. The last two visits at the hospital with the Social Worker and the Surgeon had begun to wear me down. I was not sure if I could keep struggling against both the illness and the medical community, as well as financially.

It was one evening while I was feeling dismal that I received a call from Dan, my boss. Dan has a younger brother who lives in the United States and who is a surgeon. Dan had spoken to him that day about me and that was the reason for his evening call. His voice was grave. He explained that his brother had told him I was running out of time. He felt that considering the size of my tumor and the fact that there was a second tumor in a different location, I could not afford to wait any longer. Dan said his brother had been adamant. Dan's surgeon brother thought that the natural methods would not be fast enough for me. What I needed now were The Big Guns! His brother had said that if I did not take chemotherapy immediately, The Big Gun, then I would most undoubtedly die!

That phone call came soon after my encounter with the surgeon. I had been calm in her office but her words had not been forgotten and were left in my mind where, during moments of fear, they re-appeared. And the moments of fear were increasing. I was feeling very afraid. Dan's words leaped across the telephone line and my already much-activated fear turned to sheer terror. In my mind, I had been questioning if there would be enough time to turn everything around, so Dan's words fell on very fertile ground. It was ground tilled by fear. I knew that the tumor was getting very large and growing daily, because I could feel it. It had gone from the size of a dove egg (1" x ¾" or 2 ½ x 1 ½ cm) at the end of April, to what it was now in July, barely 2 ½ months later, the size of a small grapefruit (3"x 4" or 7 x 10 cm).

While on the phone with Dan, I didn't say much. The phone conversation did not last long. Dan's reason for the call had been stated; there was no room for small talk. And when I got off the phone, I dropped my face in my hands and cried like I have never cried before. All the vigor had gone out of me, I felt like I was facing odds too overwhelming. I felt backed into a corner and could not see any way out.

Anneke entered the kitchen, where I was sitting at the table to take Dan's call. She didn't say anything but just sat down beside me. Neither one of us spoke. Finally, after what seemed like an eternity, I looked at her, feeling such despair I could hardly speak. I managed to choke out the words, "I have to take the chemo," and began to cry again. And she cried with me.

Pa and Vincent came into the kitchen, too, I told them that I had to take the chemo. It did not feel like my choice, it was still not my choice, but I was now living the surgeon's words. I felt like I was backed into a corner, that the only thing to do now was to accept the fact that I needed the "The Big Guns" (Cut, Poison and Burn), and chemotherapy was one of them. I felt defeated, deflated, that my situation was hopeless and I was very scared and I still did not want to take chemo! But I knew that I would go and take the poison at the cancer clinic. I felt that I had arrived at the end of my rope. It was a very bleak, dark evening.

We tried calling the cancer clinic that evening, but it was too late, so I called early the next day. I told them that I would come in and take the chemo. My fear became even stronger when I was given an appointment immediately. I'm not sure if they had been waiting for my call; it sure seemed that way. I do know that they are well meaning and that they do try to save people's lives. But I could not help feeling like a mouse caught in a mousetrap. I had strayed away on what, to them, was foreign territory, but now I had returned, and I was speaking their language again. I was the prodigal daughter who had returned home, and they would take me back into their fold to start chemotherapy the next day.

That evening I felt like all the healthy eating I had done had been futile. Pa asked me what I wanted to do and I told him that I wanted to eat Dutch food. So we went to a Dutch restaurant where I had a Dutch pancake filled with Dutch cheese. It was the comfort food of my childhood. Full of fat, processed flour, butter, sugar, syrup—all the foods I had not eaten in months. I thought I could just go back to eating the way I always had.

What I had not counted on was that, by now, my body

was so accustomed to eating without fat that it refused the fat and the heavy food and it was pushed out with force. I was surprised to find that I also did not enjoy it anymore. My taste buds had become quite refined, and I found this food much too sweet, too heavy and it made me feel very sluggish. As a result of eating healthy, I had never felt better. I had more energy, my skin glowed and if it had not been for the constant reminder of the large tumor growing in my left breast I felt and looked the picture of health.

Chapter Twelve

Chemotherapy

The next day, both Anneke, with her baby, and Pa came with me to the cancer clinic. The waiting room was jam-packed with people passing the time before getting chemo. I did not want to be there; I wanted to run. I did not want chemotherapy, but since I no longer felt I had a choice I meekly stayed. It was while we were sitting in the waiting room that we witnessed something incredibly insensitive. Anneke and I both saw it and, at first, we could not believe that we had actually seen what surely we must be imagining. It appalled both of us. A nurse came into the waiting room. She walked quickly to the coffee table where magazines and newspapers lay. She picked up the local newspaper, flipped through it oblivious of anyone else in the room. It was clear that she was looking for something specific. When she found the page she was looking for, she read it, put the newspaper down where she had opened it and walked out again.

Anneke and I looked at each other, with shocked faces; we asked each other, "Did you see that?" Both of us had, and we had to check with the other if what we had seen was real. It certainly was!

The nurse had picked up the obituaries! She had read them standing up in front of all of us and then returned the opened paper back to the table where it sat opened to the obituary page. We were not sure if anyone else had been aware of what had just happened. This incident revolted me, and more than ever I did not want to be there. I knew I was sharing a diagnosis with the other people in there, but I felt strongly like I did not belong in this room. I stayed, but I had to force myself not to run out of the hospital. Mutely, I waited for my turn so I could be given the poison.

Finally, it was my turn. But on my way to the Chemo room, I was intercepted by my oncologist. Before I was given chemo, he wanted to examine my breast. But instead of taking me into an examination room and giving me time to undress and put on a gown, I was taken into what seemed like a utility room and asked to lift my top so he could look at and feel my breast. It felt very invasive. I felt humiliated. It did not feel professional or even like a medical exam. It felt more like a body search at a police station done to a criminal. It felt as if this demeaning procedure was done on purpose, perhaps as a punishment for having had the nerve not to follow his recommended treatment.

Since I had temporarily lost my voice and my courage, due to stress, fear, and exhaustion I did not speak up for myself to protest and insist to be taken into a proper examination room. He was very brusque and his kindly gentle bedside manner was nowhere to be found. I felt like I was treated without respect or kindness, very much like a number. And even though Anneke and Pa had come to the hospital with me, I was not given a choice to have them come into the room with me. The reason given was that it would be a very quick examination—again at their convenience and at my expense. To cater to this huge industry at a time when I needed support, I was not even allowed to have the familiar presence of my family during this invasive examination. This time it was not my choice to be alone. I had months ago realized that I needed human comfort and support during this difficult time. Today, as if to confirm that I didn't have a choice, I was not offered an option. I had to endure this alone.

After this degrading examination, I was taken into a room by an intern and she measured the tumor and recorded the numbers. It was now official: It was very large and measured 3" x 4" or 7 x 10 cm. Another lump was found under my left armpit in the lymph node and measured at 1 ½" or 4 cm. This was stage III cancer.

After all this, I was finally taken to what I call The Chemo room. It was a large, open area where people were sitting on reclining hospital chairs hooked up to IV poles. Some were chatting to each other, as if they were at a tea party. Others just sat staring into space. To me, it was an awful room. I was assigned one of the green chairs and asked to sit down. Then I, too, was hooked up to an IV, and the bag holding the chemo was placed on the IV pole. It began to drip, and I could feel it go into my veins; it felt ice-cold and heavy. I was trying to be brave, but when I looked over at the other people in the room and saw a young woman with a "funny" hat telling another woman that she lost her hair before she returned for her next treatment, I began to cry softly. The accumulated stress and the recently endured attacks by the oncologist, the surgeon, and the social worker, had seriously depleted my courage. I did not want this. I had not asked for any of this.

I did not want the cancer, and I certainly did not want the chemo. I looked at Anneke and I gave voice to my thoughts that I did not want any of it. She just nodded, unable to speak: She knew! We just sat there, not knowing what else to say. I was glad for her presence; my sister, my friend, we who normally never stopped talking when we were together, silenced by what was happening now.

After about 45 minutes, less than an hour, it was over and my body was now filled with a poison to kill the malignant cells which had created tumors. I felt like the old lady who had swallowed a fly. Like me and the chemo, she swallowed a spider to catch the fly, would she die? Then she swallowed all the other animals to catch the smaller ones etc., when finally she died, not from the fly, but from having swallowed all the other animals to catch the fly. Would I too die from the spider swallowed to catch the fly, from this poison? I was not sure of anything at this point.

We went home, but not before I was given pills costing $20 each. They were anti-nausea pills. I was given a prescription for a three-day supply, to be taken as needed for nausea. I had no Medical Plan; I made only $1600 a month, from which I had to pay a mortgage, a student loan, car loan payments, and try to survive on the rest. I also had to buy expensive organic food, vitamins, supplements, food, and school supplies for my 14-year-old son. I certainly did not have several hundred dollars to cover the cost for a three day supply of expensive $20 pills—anti nausea medication. It turned out that the nurses have what they call a *black market* supply from which they can dispense pills for free when someone cannot afford to buy them. Surprisingly, somehow, I did qualify for this service. Of course I was now following the recommended treatment, and with that came financial support.

And so I left with my expensive free *black market* supply of anti nausea pills. I had taken one before the chemo treatment, but before we got home it was already becoming apparent that they were not going to work for me. I was beginning to feel very very nauseous.

I did not feel like being sick with a house full of people around me. I wanted to be by myself, so I sent everyone, including Vincent, away. He went for an overnight visit with family. And while everyone was away I felt sicker than I have ever felt at any other time in my life. The rest of the afternoon, I either spent in the bathroom on my knees in front of the toilet vomiting or on my way to it. I had suffered morning sickness 24 hours a day during my pregnancy with Vincent. That seemed like mere queasiness compared to the extreme nausea I was now experiencing.

It was during one of my episodes on the floor in the bathroom that I heard an incredible clatter. There was a loud pounding sound on the roof as if thousands of machine guns were being fired at it. Was it the outbreak of a war? I had no idea what could be making such noise. I got up fast and ran to the window to see what it was.

What I had not realized while kneeling in front of my toilet

111

was that a storm of storms was raging outside. It was the fiercest summer storm I have ever witnessed. It was hail with thunder and ferocious winds. So much hail fell that afternoon that my entire little emerging garden was completely and utterly destroyed. Before the storm, my neighbors across the street had a beautiful flower garden; after the storm all that was left were very short sad looking stubbly stems. Nature was showing its dominance that day and in its wake left a path of destruction. Not only were gardens destroyed, tree branches were torn off, and entire trees were ripped out by their roots. Nature ravaged not only itself but many manmade structures. Every house in the neighborhood needed its roof replaced: Awnings, siding, and windows were all destroyed,

So much hail fell, it looked like winter. The hail piled up deeply against my house and, since there was no frost (after all, it was summer), it began to leak into my basement. A lot of damage had been done by nature in less than an hour.

I could not help feeling that this might be a reflection of what was happening inside my body. Was it a parallel to what was being destroyed inside my body? *Evil* cells as well as healthy cells? I do know that my body aged greatly that day. I would discover that when my hair grew back. My entire head would be covered with silver gray, almost white, hair. I was only 38! Before the chemo treatment I had a few gray hairs, but certainly not that much. At 38, I was considered to be in the summer of my life, but when my hair returned almost white, it made me look as if I were in the winter of my life. I had the hair color of an old woman.

That day of the chemo and the summer hail storm, I still felt very nauseous, but I also realized that something larger, outside of me, was happening. Was God reminding me that He was there? I would not have heard a whisper or even a voice yelling. I would only have paid attention to a roar. And this hailstorm was roaring. It was nature at its loudest, its destruction extreme. I felt very much a part of something larger. I knew I belonged in this universe and that we could plan all we want; we could try to grow beautiful gardens, tend to them, water them, but they could be destroyed in a heartbeat by the force of nature. That's exactly what happened on July 16, 1996.

My garden had been hit hard, but it was not destroyed permanently. As early as the next day, some of the plants began to lift themselves back up. Others were too broken and did not return until the next year, but their roots were strong. And even though my garden was torn and battered, it was slowly recovering and starting to come back to life. I feel that my garden represents me, especially when I look outside today and see how lush and green and healthy my little garden is. Yes, that day in July, my plants seemed destroyed and crushed, the same way my immune system was seemingly destroyed and crushed as a result of the chemo. But despite the destruction we both suffered, both my garden and I are still here today—not just hanging in there, barely surviving, but stronger and more vibrant than ever.

That day, in the summer of '96, was a dark day, indeed. The next day, Vincent returned. I was still feeling quite ill. The expensive pills, which were supposed to have combatted the dreaded side effect of chemotherapy, nausea, had not helped me at all.

Chapter Thirteen

Hair: Look good, feel good...

The nausea stayed with me almost 3 days, but when I was able to eat again, I resumed eating healthy food and taking supplements. The days were busy with work, reading, and focusing on life. After the chemo/hailstorm day, the routine of life and concentrating on staying alive swiftly took hold of me again. Two weeks went by quickly. Then came the morning in the shower—I was washing my hair, when I looked down and noticed far more hair on the floor of my bathtub than was usual. I touched my hair and looked at my fingers: They were covered in hair. I pulled very gently on some hair and, to my horror, I could feel them detaching from my scalp. My hair was no longer strongly attached to my head. My hair was beginning to fall out!

I had always had thick long hair, but now one after the other it was as if my hairs were releasing themselves from my scalp. Standing there in the shower, I realized that the chemotherapy treatment's other awful side effect was beginning to manifest itself. I was loosing my hair, but maybe, I hoped, I would not lose all my hair. Maybe I would only lose some of my hair and not become totally bald. I wanted to weep, but I tried to suppress the tears because I had to get ready for work; no time for crying now. But I was feeling so miserable. I am a woman and, as most women know, we are very connected with our hair, and I wanted to keep mine. But time was ticking; I could not afford the luxury of dwelling on my misery: I had to get ready to go to work so I wouldn't be late. I quickly dressed, but I was afraid to comb or touch my hair. Maybe, if I left it alone, it would stop falling out.

In the midst of getting ready and trying to fend off despair, with a jolt I remembered a dream I had about a year earlier. In the dream, I was standing in the shower; I remembered reaching over to put shampoo in my hair. It seemed, in that dream, that I had thought that there was something in the shampoo, something that affected my hair, because cleaning it caused all my hair to fall out and rain down into the drain. By the end of the dream, I had no hair left—I was bald.

But this was no dream; this was real, and my hair was really falling out. I was hoping that maybe I had only imagined it because everyone knows that chemotherapy makes you lose your hair; I was hoping, desperately, that somehow the chemo had not affected me that way. I had to check again, so very gently I pulled at a few to assure myself I had only imagined what I had seen earlier in the shower. But horror of horror, it happened again. Once more I felt the hair shafts releasing the hair from my scalp.

So far, this had been a very hard journey; but this—this was such a hard blow. I did not know how I could bear this. I did not want to lose my hair, I did not want to be bald, and I did not want to wear funny little hats or fashionable turbans. When I see someone wearing any of these, I immediately think, "There goes a cancer patient," and I did not want to be identified as a cancer patient.

I wanted to wake up; I wanted all of it to go away. I wanted a genie to come out of my shampoo bottle and shake her head or wiggle her nose and send all my hair flying back onto my scalp to reattach themselves so I could have my long thick hair back. I wanted to scream at God; I wanted to run to my mother. But my mother was not here, and the reality I would have to face was that I would lose all my hair.

Normally, I dry my hair forcefully with a towel; that morning

I sort of patted it dry, still hardly touching it at all. Even with that, a lot of hair fell on the floor. When it had air-dried I, oh so carefully, combed my hair, barely touching it at all. Still, many hairs stayed behind on the comb, and I noticed that now some were on my shoulder, as well. I tried not to panic: If I could only think of something else, then it would not seem so bad. But I felt sheer terror at the thought of not having any hair, of being bald!

I did not want to think about my hair and what was happening with it anymore, so I tried to take special care with my make-up and what I wore that morning. But it was to no avail when all I could really think about was my hair. I liked having long thick hair, and I wanted to keep it that way—but it looked like that was not going to happen. Everything pointed to the fact that I would lose my hair. The only thing I did not yet know, that morning, was how long it would take before I lost all my hair, or whether I would lose all of my hair.

I had to leave and go to my office, where everyone had been very supportive and kind. Absentmindedly, I drove to work. When I got there and stepped out of my car, I looked at the driver's seat, and I was shocked. The entire seat on the driver's side was covered with long blonde hairs. My hair! I did not even try to clean them off, but quickly turned away from the sight; I tried very hard not to look at this new horror. Maybe if I ignored it, it would all go away?

Blinking away my tears, which were so close to the surface, I walked through the outside door into the reception area. I had tried so hard to be brave since my dreadful discovery in the shower. As I walked in, Sherron, our receptionist, asked how I was, and at that moment my already shaky resolve crumbled. I looked at her and all I could choke out was, "I'm losing my hair!" And then I finally cried!

I don't know how she had left her desk and how she had moved so quickly, but there she was holding me, while together we cried over my hair, the cancer, and the unfairness of it all. This was not supposed to happen. Women are not supposed to get breast cancer and lose their hair. Strangers do, but not me.

Yet here I was, trying to fight courageously to stay alive, doing all I could to survive this deadly foe, giving up luxuries so I could eat healthy and pay for supplements. And now, on top of that, I was losing my hair. None of what had occurred previously had affected me on the outside. The fight was mostly taking place internally—inside my body, inside my mind, inside my emotions. But the loss of my hair was the first external manifestation and, for me, that was my lowest point. It was as if this was the straw that had now broken the camel's back.

But as difficult as this moment, this mountain on my road, was, deep inside I knew I would overcome this, too. I would face it and do what I had to do. I would wear a wig, so that only people I chose to tell would know what I was battling. That's how I wanted it to be. I would not wear funny, strange hats or fashionable turbans. I would look as normal as other people. I would not let myself be visibly identified as a cancer patient.

In 1996, not too many healthy people were shaving their heads yet in support of cancer. Even with that, people who shave their heads still have their eyebrows and eyelashes. I would be lucky, my lashes would only thin out, and I would not lose them all. And I did not lose any eyebrow hairs at all. Losing any other body hair on the parts normally covered by clothes was not a big deal to me. That at least stayed hidden.

Earlier, during Anneke's visit, she and I had been to the cancer support center where they also have a wig lending library. Knowing about chemo therapy's hair loss side effect, we had both tried on wigs. We had tried to act silly and lighthearted, but the ever present threat made it difficult to be care-free. We tried to cover it by trying on outrageous hair pieces. The first wig I had tried on had long red hair. It looked horrible. The woman there had told us that almost every woman wants to try on a red wig. I quickly realized what a mistake this was for me. Red hair does not go at all with my skin color, and the long straight style may have looked right for me when I was a teenager, it did absolutely nothing for me now.

I thought that most of the wigs in the lending library available that day were very ugly. They looked like wigs, with exaggerated styles and curls: even the most dimwitted person could easily identify them as fake hairpieces. I had picked up two, anyway, just in case, even though, against all odds, I had hoped I would be spared the ordeal of losing my hair. Both of them were short, one was curly and one straight, and I hated them equally. They were "fuddy duddy" hairstyles and they looked frumpy. I didn't want to wear them. They made me feel ugly. The last thing I wanted to do was feel ugly. This disease was already attacking how I felt about myself as a woman; it was attacking my breast and now my hair, too, was being attacked. I felt very let down by my own body—could it not hold on to the one thing I knew that had always been one of my assets: my hair?

I wanted to keep my own hair, at least until my next chemo appointment. I wanted in defiance to show *Them* at the cancer clinic that I got to keep my hair. In my mind, I called the mainstream medical community *Them* because I did not feel like we were on the same side; I felt very much like we were a divided *Them* and *Us*. But every day I woke up and found my pillow and my bed covered in hair. If I drove somewhere, my car and the driver's seat were covered in hair. My couch, my chair, my house, everything was covered in hair. I had not realized how much hair grows on a human head. With the large amount I had already lost, I should have been bald, but I was not. Not yet, I was given a bit of a reprise because I still did not look like a cancer patient. I was still presentable, but by now my hair was getting very thin. I had never been able to see my scalp show through my hair, but now I could see pink skin shine through.

The day when I would be given the next dose of chemo arrived. This time, Irene, my rowing buddy, came with me. We waited together in the waiting room. By now, I had become accustomed to waiting and knew it appeared to be an inevitable evil associated with the cancer clinic. The nurse came and called my name; it was my turn. She took me to the large hall, The Chemo room! It was a room I remembered all too well from July 16. What an industry! People came in and went out in a few hours. I was amazed at the sheer number of people I kept seeing at the cancer clinic. So many people appeared to be sick with this disease.

Just like before, I was taken to a chair so I could be hooked up again to the IV pole with the poison. But just before I sat down and before the nurse had a chance to 'hook' me up in my designated chair, a part of me spoke up again. I had not known what I would say, or what I would do. I had not planned anything. I thought I had come to the cancer clinic to take the next dose, yet it was as if another part of me was in charge again. I almost felt as if I could observe myself when I told her I wanted to see my doctor. It was my voice; it was me who asked, but what was I going to say? The nurse looked a little taken aback, but she did not argue with me before she escorted me into an examining room. Before she left, she asked me to put on a gown and went to find the doctor. After only a short wait, she returned with a young intern. I asked the young female doctor what they had been expecting from the chemo. She answered, "We were hoping for some shrinkage [of the tumor]."

"It has," I answered her. And I instructed her by saying, "I want you to measure it."

She took out a measuring tape and did just that: She agreed that it had shrunk. "However," she added, "only somewhat." I knew this was an understatement and that it had shrunk a lot more than somewhat.

Again, as if someone else was in charge of my voice, I heard myself saying to her that I was not going to have another dose of chemo. I was not taking any more. The young female doctor told me this was against her advice and that this was not wise. But I calmly repeated my statement. She looked at me gravely and said, perhaps to try and change my mind, "You better be scared, if your doctors are scared."

I looked directly into her eyes, when I replied firmly, "Do you think I am not scared, do you think that I don't know what this is? Because I do, and I am scared, but I am not having any more chemotherapy. And now I want to schedule my surgery."

She must, at that point have realized that I meant what I was saying. "O. K.," she said. "We will contact your surgeon and set it up, and she mentioned the name of the angry surgeon I had consulted earlier in the summer." No!' I answered, "I don't want that surgeon! I would like you to give me names of other surgeons."

I didn't give her a reason why I wanted another surgeon, and she did not ask. But my reason for this request was that I felt that anyone who was as angry with me, as my first surgeon had been, at my perceived *dictating* of my own treatment, would not be beneficial for me. I certainly did not want her to operate on me, when I was helpless and under general anesthetic. The intern said she would have the nurse give me names of other surgeons. And with that she left the room.

The nurse gave me names, and she told me about one doctor in particular who had operated on her mother. I placed him at the top of my list. I felt that nurses would choose someone they felt comfortable with and about whom they knew would do a good job on their mothers. And then the nurse told me something, for which I am still very grateful. She looked at me and said, "I hope you find something!" And she continued by saying, "Because cancer is increasing. It is an epidemic!" She then quoted the figures, "One in three people would get cancer in a lifetime." There were three of us in that little room that day: Irene and I and the nurse. This time, I was the designated cancer patient. Lucky them! But would they escape the curse? Or would they be in another group of three, when it would be their turn to be the designated cancer patient?

It was what she told me next that encouraged me. She told me that years ago, one of her friends, a nurse, had been diagnosed with a very aggressive stomach cancer. She, because of her profession, knew the types of traditional treatments available, and chose not to use any. She was too aware of the health risks associated with each of the three. The nurse's face showed deep emotions as she told me the story of her friend who had chosen alternative methods. I waited to hear the negative message I was expecting but, instead, to my surprise, I heard the nurse tell me that her friend is not only alive, she is cancer free. This happened 10 years ago. I thanked her for having told me this; we smiled at each other and Irene and I left. I had just received a wonderful life affirming story from one of *Them*. But by presenting me with this gift, the line between *Them* (Mainstream Medical Community) and *Us* (anything to do with Alternative Methods) was not so fixed anymore.

The day I had gone to the cancer clinic was my last good hair day. Somehow, I had met the stubborn promise I had made to myself to show *Them* I had not lost my hair. But, now, it was very obvious that my hair loss was continuing and that in a very short time I would be completely bald. Some people, when they reach this point, cut their hair short or shave it as soon as they begin to realize that their hair is falling out. The reason for this is twofold: First, somehow the hair loss seems less traumatic when you lose short stubbles; the second reason is that cutting their hair gives people some measure of control: They now decide when and where they lose their hair. I have almost always had long hair, so even cutting it shorter would be traumatic for me.

But I could no longer ignore the fact I had to do something with my disappearing hair. Since the wigs from the cancer support center were so ugly, my family had offered to buy me a wig. That afternoon, I was going to a hair salon that sold wigs. So, together with Jenni and Pa, we went to a local mall, where I would try and find a wig I liked. Pa and Jenni were there to offer me support and help me decide on a wig. By now, my hair was very, very thin. I had been afraid to wash it. During the last days I had barely combed it and touched it even less; yet, it had continued to fall out in clumps. It felt like my house and my car had grown hair. There were hairs everywhere—everywhere but on my head.

The hair salon had an immense selection of wigs, and even though some looked very much like wigs, many looked natural and some were quite beautiful. There was one in particular that had caught my eye. It not only looked natural, but when I tried it on, it looked like my own hair, and I knew this was the one for me. It was made with real hair and the color and highlights looked very much like my disappearing hair; even the length of

121

this wig was almost identical to the length I usually wore my hair at.

The hairdresser looked after many people with hair loss from cancer treatment, and his empathic behavior was very calming. Everyone in that hair salon was very kind and gentle, without being patronizing. They were also respectful, trying to ease my experience as much as possible. Before the hairdresser shaped and trimmed the wig, he washed my hair. The shaping and trimming of the wig would be done while it was on my head. I did not want to look at my face in the mirror, but I was surrounded by my own reflection and could not help seeing myself.

When I looked at the woman in the chair, I saw a cancer patient. Large patches of my skull were now hairless, and only thin clumps of hair remained. I felt like a freak. In the mirror's reflection, I could see Pa's face behind me and I saw that seeing me like that was hard for him too. But beside Pa, I saw Jenni's smiling face, and I was grateful for her calming, serene presence, both for me and Pa.

While trying to fight back tears and trying to come to terms with the picture of myself in the mirror, I had not looked at the woman in the chair beside me. But she, of course, had noticed me. I became aware of her when she gently spoke to me. I looked at her in the mirror when she asked me if I was being treated for cancer. I wanted to say, "Isn't it obvious?", but answered her with only "Yes." She asked kindly with tender concern, "Breast cancer?" I nodded.

She continued to speak and said to me, "I've had it too." She then said, "I had a double mastectomy and have had replacement surgery." She now had my full attention, and I turned in my chair to look at her fully, no longer looking in the mirror at her image but really looking at her, instead. We smiled at each other, and then she asked me, "Would you like to see my new breasts?" The conversation was somewhat surreal, yet felt as normal, as if we were talking about a piece of jewelry instead of body parts. I realized that I very much wanted to see her *new* breasts. I wanted to see what breast construction looked like, so again I nodded.

And there we were, strangers on this journey of life, yet bound by a dreadful disease. Together, we walked to the back, where my wig was being washed in a small room. The woman, whose name I did not even know, asked if we could be alone in the little room for a moment. When it was just her and me, she calmly opened her blouse and showed me her perfect replacement pair of breasts. She explained that she did not yet have any new nipples, but told me that these too would be added later. They would even have color added, much like a tattoo. As surreal as the moment had earlier felt, it now felt incredibly real. I was connecting with someone who had walked the same path I was currently on, and she had survived the ordeal. She looked beautiful and confident and wonderfully human. It helped me immensely to meet her: That day, I do believe she had been sent to help me, to make the journey a little easier for me. Meeting her helped to allow me to see light at the end of the tunnel, on that dark day when I became hairless for a while.

I do not recall what else we talked about in that small back room; remembering it now, it once more seems somewhat surreal. Yet, I think about her sometimes. Is she still doing well? How do her new nipples look? What is her name? I don't remember her face, but I do remember her neat beautiful *new* breasts, and her kindness in showing me such an intimate part of herself. Our lives briefly touched and mine was richer for it. We walked out of the small room together, and I no longer felt as vulnerable. An encounter with a stranger had left me stronger and had reminded me this, too, shall pass.

I sat back down in my chair, and beside me appeared the hairdresser with my now dry wig. Before he put it on to style it, he cut whatever hair was remaining on my head, very short. I didn't want to look at myself; I looked so alien, so foreign to myself, yet I was unable to tear my eyes away from the image in the mirror. But this time, I could look at myself with renewed strength, with renewed resolve, with the knowledge that this was temporary.

It was still weird—was that strange looking creature really me? I watched what was happening to me, with detached fascination. Is that the mind's way of having us deal with shock and stress? Or was it because I had become calm from my encounter with a kind stranger? As if it were someone else's head, I looked at my skull and noticed that it has a nice shape. Somehow, with the very short hair, it did not look as awful as it had with long hair and many patches missing. With short hair, it was not as noticeable that much of my skull was showing, and it no longer seemed so awful, either.

But I was used to myself with long hair. I liked long hair. And I was very grateful that my *new* hair, the wig, was long. And so, when he placed the wig on my head, I recognized myself again. It was a beautiful wig, shoulder length, with bangs and highlights. The hairdresser began to shape it to compliment my face; he trimmed and cut and it looked great. Actually, my own hair had never looked this good. My own hair had always had a mind of its own. This style was sleek and sophisticated. I felt pretty and, somehow, not so lost anymore. By now, everyone in the hair salon had turned his or her attention to me. It was not just a wig place, and people were coming and going having all sorts of things done to their hair. It was busy, yet the focus of the entire place was completely on what was happening to me. Short of cheering loudly, everyone there gave me the thumbs up, telling me how good it looked. Yet I could tell my presence had affected people deeply, and I saw tears glistening in many eyes. But I was feeling great with my new hair and I could see how good it looked from my image in the mirror. I looked at where Jenni and my dad were sitting, and I could see both of them smiling broadly.

When I came home, I called out to Vincent. I asked him how he liked my hair. He looked up from what he was doing and glanced briefly at my head, the way 14 year old boys do when their mothers have a new hairstyle, and mumbled, "Nice haircut mom."

"It's not a haircut Vincent," I said. "It's a wig." He turned to look at it in amazement and said, "It looks just like your own hair!" And, strangely, it was true: As much as it was sleeker and a more sophisticated style, it did look very much like my own hair. The color was very similar to the hair I had just lost, and even the texture was quite similar.

That evening, I wanted to test my wig, so I drove to another local mall. I wanted to see what it felt like to go out in public. Would people stare and point and say, "Look at that woman wearing a wig?" Would they look away in obvious embarrassment? None of that happened; no one seemed to be looking at me strangely. And even though that night was very windy, the wig did not fly off. It stayed snugly on my head. Weeks later, I would even go horseback riding and, even then, the wig did not come off. They really do make marvelous wigs these days. How comforting for cancer patients and other people who need to wear wigs for other reasons.

The next day, I went to my office to show off my new hair to my bosses and co-workers. There, too, I was met with great enthusiasm and lots of compliments about how good I looked with my new temporary hair. Since I was eating very healthy, with not much fat in my diet as an added bonus, I was losing weight. I could see in the mirror that I looked great; I was becoming quite slim. But having a head full of thick, healthy looking hair, again, lifted my spirits immensely.

A few days later, I went to an afternoon at the Canadian cancer Society. It was for the *Look Good, Feel Good* presentation. I already knew what a difference wearing a wig had made for me. What I didn't realize was how emotional it would be for me to see and hear other women dealing with this disease. Some, like me, were wearing wigs. Others still had their hair, and still others were wearing hats and turbans. But we were all battling the same disease: cancer. That afternoon, we laughed, we cried and again, strangers gave me comfort. Many professionals were volunteering their time, and companies had donated a variety of make-up articles. The make-up was enough to last me for months.

My main reason for going had been to receive the free products. Since buying the vitamins and eating organic food had not left me with any spare money for luxuries, such as make-up, I had to be resourceful and find a way to get some beauty products. This had been my answer. But I received much more than free stuff. I received human comfort and laughter. Wearing make-up and feeling good was healing for me, but being with others who were fighting the same battle, hearing their stories and telling mine, made me feel not quite so alone.

Chapter Fourteen

Surgery

Time passed, and we were now at the beginning of September. My surgery date was not until September 20. This time was needed for me to get strong and recover from the chemotherapy. I continued with the supplements, eating organically and including lots of vegetables and fruit in my diet, seeing Dr. Jones for immune boosting treatments and meeting with Julie for Psychosynthesis. During the Psychosynthesis sessions I was discovering more and more about myself.

I was also continuing with my visits every other day to Dr. Jones, my chiropractor. The support all these people gave me cannot be measured by money. After all, I am alive: What is the value of a life? Can it be measured by money? The person I am: Vincent's mother, Pa's daughter, my siblings' sister, many people's friend. If you were to ask any of them what they would pay to keep me alive, what would their answer be? Would they give all they have, and would that be enough? So, how do you place a monetary value on a life? It is not possible.

After receiving names of surgeons, I began to interview them. The first doctor I interviewed was the one at the top of my list. He was the person who had operated on the nurse's mother. Once again, Jenni had come with me for support and to write down answers and ask questions. This man took lots of time to explain his method of surgery. He not only talked to me at length, he also listened to and answered all my questions. At one point during the conversation, I looked at him and said, "Thank you for treating me like an intelligent human being."

"Well, you are," he answered.

"I know that," I replied, "but I have not felt that I have been treated like an intelligent woman by your colleagues."

I felt at ease with this man, something which was very important to me. I then asked the surgeon how long I had to stay in the hospital.

"We usually keep you a few days," he said, "but if you want to leave earlier, you can." I was being given a choice and it felt very empowering.

"What about hospital food" I asked, "Do I have to eat it?"

"Not at all," he replied, "If you want to bring your own food, that's up to you."

I knew that I would let this man operate my tumor, and I told him so. We then scheduled the surgery date. After we left his office, both Jenni and I shared our mutual liking of this very human surgeon.

Sept. 20: My surgery date had finally arrived. Vincent and Pa had taken me to the hospital and we were now sitting together in the waiting room. Patients who came in for surgery were all waiting there with their families. When their time came, they would walk to the operating room, accompanied by their loved ones. The family and friends would wait outside the door until surgery was finished. Earlier, I had been given a gown and a housecoat. I was also wearing slippers. We did not talk much, the three of us; conversation is not easy when you are facing a cancer operation.

I had earlier seen my surgeon speaking with another patient, but now he walked back into the waiting room and he approached us. He sat down beside me and began to explain what would happen that day. He explained that he would cut as small as possible around the tumor. It would then be sent to the lab, while I was still unconscious from the anesthetic. I would lay waiting on the operating table. If there was a clear margin, he would stop. A clear margin means there are no cancer cells in the area around the tumor. If, however, he found cancer cells, he would cut small again making the radius where the tumor had been a little larger. With me still under anesthetics, it would again be sent to the lab, where again they would check for cancer cells. And this would continue until no cancer cells were found, until he found the desired clear margin. He explained that this could take all day, but he would continue to cut small so that I would lose as little as possible of my breast. However, he warned me there was still a possibility I could wake up and find it had been necessary to take my entire breast. I was going into an unknown, and I would wake up to an unknown. It was possible that I would wake up after a full mastectomy was performed on me. Not a very reassuring thought. But I appreciated his honesty.

My surgery time had arrived, and it was time for Vincent and my dad to walk me to the door. I could tell by their faces this was a very difficult walk for them, as it was for me. We did not know what the surgeon would find, and I could wake up to a devastating loss. Saying goodbye at an airport to a dear friend or a loved relative is difficult, but saying goodbye to your mother and daughter who is about to enter going into an operating room, being operated for cancer, must be almost intolerable. I can only imagine, by the look on their faces, how difficult that moment was for both of them.

My father is a large man. My son was on the threshold of manhood, but seeing them standing there, both looking very helpless, almost broke my heart. I would have given anything for them not to have to face this. Standing on the sideline, helplessly, while a loved one faces something of this magnitude and not being able to do anything but be there, is one of the hardest things we as human beings face. It was difficult for me, but at least I could do something. I could fight—they could only stand powerlessly looking on from the sidelines and watch and wait and pray.

As I opened the door, I looked back one more time at my teenage son and my senior father before I walked into the operating area. The doors closed behind me with a thud.

In the area behind the doors there were some chairs. I walked towards them and sat down; a woman I had seen earlier was already sitting there. I had seen her in the main waiting area where she had sat on the opposite side of the room. We waited side by side on those chairs while nurses brought us warmed blankets for our feet. Next, in preparation for our surgery, it was time for us to put little, ugly, paper caps on our head. Before I put the paper cap on I took my wig off, and the stranger beside me gasped a little. She told me that she had been looking at me in the waiting room and had been admiring my hair. I smiled, held up the wig, and jokingly said, "You too, can have hair like this." As we both laughed, we exchanged names. Today, I cannot remember her name, but she was to remember mine. The next time I saw her, after my surgery, she told me that when I was waking up in the recovery room, her surgery had finished earlier and she was already fully awake. She heard the nurses call me Margaret, before I woke up, but she explained to them that my name was really Margreet. This was a good thing, because I have always disliked being called Margaret. It is a fine name for others, but I am Margreet.

After a short waiting time, a nurse walked me into the operating room where I was asked to lie down on the operating table. Other nurses were busying themselves with equipment when the Anesthesiologist came in. He was about to give me anesthetics when I told him I had a question for him. He stopped what he was doing and looked at me quizzically, ready to hear my question.

"Have you been drinking?" I asked him. I heard a nurse's intake of breath and I could see that another one was about to break into laughter. He looked at me puzzled.

"I had orange juice," he said. It was about 11 am.

"No," I replied, "I mean alcohol: Have you been drinking alcohol?" This time one of the nurses did laugh out loud, thinking it to be a joke. It wasn't: I was quite serious. He must have realized the significance because he answered me in the same vein and answered me that no, he had not been drinking.

Then he proceeded to tell the nurses that this was not really such a strange question, after all. When he was an intern, he had been called to assist a doctor who had to listen to a young woman's heart. This doctor had forgotten his stethoscope and so he listened with his ear placed on the young woman's chest. Because he had been quite inebriated he had fallen asleep on her upper body.

Hearing his tale, we all laughed. The nurses had shifted their focus momentarily from readying the equipment, and we had all shared in the funny story. I realized that because of this humorous exchange, I was no longer a patient: I had become a person with a voice and with a mind. What a different experience from the time when I had my first biopsy taken, in that other room with those cold women. Today, in this operating room, we had shared laughter and a life story. It made me feel a little stronger, knowing that they saw my humanity before I was to slip into unconsciousness from the anesthetics.

My question had not been random. I had a reason for asking this question: In 1980, I had read a newspaper article about an anesthesiologist who had a serious drinking problem. He was often inebriated when performing his task and was usually able to cover up. However, the article had been written about him because one day he had not been able to cover up a serious mistake in the dose he had administered to a patient, and the person had died as a result—definitely a case of iatrogenic (doctor induced) death. He practiced at the hospital where my surgery was being performed. It was something that I had never forgotten, and this was the reason I had asked the anesthesiologist a seeminly odd question.

When next the surgeon entered, I asked him too if he had been drinking. This time it was a joke! I had a sense about this doctor. My impressions of him made me feel quite certain that he would not go into surgery having consumed any alcohol. The nurses and the anesthesiologist all laughed when I asked the question again. We were laughing together. The general mood in that operating room was, somehow, a little lighter. The reason we were there was serious, but the laughter had changed the mood in the room. Laughter, it is said, is not a bad beginning and certainly not a bad ending. It was healing for me and good for the energy in that room. Next, while I still had a smile on my face, I was asked to count backwards from 100, and before I got to 95 I was asleep, with a hint of laughter still in the air.

My next memory is waking up with an excruciating pain in my left breast. It felt like someone had used a very sharp knife and cut into my chest. That is what it felt like and, of course, that is exactly what had happened. But did I still have my breast? That was my first conscious thought. I did not yet have command over my voice, so I could not ask the nurses. I drifted in and out of consciousness. I was trying to wake up, use my voice and ask that question, but I could not make a sound. Still drifting in and out of consciousness, I thought I saw the surgeon come into the room through a fog. I strained to wake up: I wanted to ask him, I wanted to talk, but I could barely see him. And then it seemed that in this dream-like state, I heard him say, "Good news, we have a clear margin!" But I was not sure if I was actually awake or dreaming. Was he real or part of a dream?

I had not realized the full extent of the importance that piece of information held for me. But my body knew. Hearing what he said or what I thought he had said, I began to gasp for air and could not catch my breath. I was still not fully alert and yet thinking I heard those words, I began to hyperventilate. But had the surgeon been real; had he actually walked into the recovery room and talked to me? Had he really said to me, "We have a clear margin" or was he a hallucination, a cruel figment of my own imagination? Was I so desperate for those words that I was dreaming them up? I could still not talk and now, on top of that, a nurse placed an oxygen mask over my face to help regulate my breathing. The nurses could tell I was trying to talk but with the oxygen mask over my face, they encouraged me not to. But I had to speak because I still had a very important question I desperately needed answering. I did not know whether I still had a breast left, and if so, how much of it was still there or, worse, how little?

I gave up trying to talk; I just had to be patient a little while longer. I allowed myself to calm down and let the drowsiness wear off gradually. Having no sense of time, I was finally wheeled into a hospital room. It was a semi-private room, which was very nice. I did not have any medical insurance, but another nice stranger at the admission desk had made sure that I was taken to a semi-private room at no extra charge. She told me that all other rooms were full. I found out, soon, that this was not entirely true. Minutes after I had arrived in my room, the woman I had spoken to earlier, right before my operation, walked into my room. She was wearing pajamas, slippers, and a housecoat, and was holding her IV pole. She exclaimed, "So here you are!" As if I was a long lost friend. She told me that she had been searching for me because she wanted to know how I was. As soon as she was able, she had walked from room to room trying to find me. We had connected as human beings while waiting for our surgeries, and she came to find out how I was and to offer comfort.

She, who had just had a gallstone operation of her own, looked full of concern for me. Hours earlier, we had not even known each other's names; we were now no longer strangers. She came to bring me human support. It gave me a warm, nurturing feeling.

After she asked me how I was feeling, she became aware of my room; she looked around and told me that she had insurance and had asked for a semi-private room. Admitting had told her that no semi-private rooms were available. "Is anyone in that other bed," she asked me. I didn't' think there was and she asked if I would mind if she came and stayed in the room with me. I didn't mind; in fact, it felt nice to see a kind, somewhat familiar face. She was about the age my mother had been when she died, and her manner was very motherly towards me. She left to enquire and returned shortly with an orderly carrying her things. She sat on the bed, and she told me that she had been in the recovery room with me and that they had called me Margaret, but she had corrected them, and told them that my name was Margreet.

When I had first been wheeled into the room, I had been feeling drowsy, but when she told me that she had been in the recovering room with me, I was instantly more awake. I realized that she had been there while I was regaining consciousness. I could ask her my burning question. Maybe she would be able to give me an answer to it.

"Did you see my surgeon there; did my surgeon come into the recovery room to see me?" I asked eagerly.

She said she thought she had seen someone dressed for surgery, but because she did not know him she was not sure. When I asked her if she remembered what he had said to me, she said she could not be sure, and didn't know. I felt deflated; I still did not have an answer to what I so desperately needed to know. While we were still talking about him, the door opened and there stood my surgeon, smiling! Surely that was a good sign? He was still dressed in surgical gear. It was only a few feet from the door to my bed but it seemed as if once again time slowed before he reached the side of my bed. He moved closely to my bed before he spoke, but then he announced, "Good news! We have a clear margin!"

Relief rushed through me and, instantly, my eyes flooded with tears. But he had not delivered all his good news yet: He continued, "And the tumor was only 1. 9cm." I felt tension I did not even realize I had ease from my body, but I still needed to ask something else. I did not know everything yet, did not completely understand the full significance of what he was telling me. Whatever the answer would be, I needed to know the whole truth. So, apprehensively, I asked, "Do I still have my breast?"

"Yes"! He affirmed with a nod and a smile. "We were able to remove your tumor by performing a lumpectomy." I know he said more, but all I heard was "Yes!"

One little word, and yet it created such a powerful impact on my spirit! "The surgery was a success," he resumed, "and your lymph nodes were clean." I wanted to laugh, I wanted to cry, but suddenly I felt very tired—not just tired, but weary and utterly exhausted. The walk on that long road, forcibly started on Sunday April 30, 1996, was almost coming to an end. I had fought very hard, and now I felt very worn out. I had run a marathon to save my life; now, I was almost at the finish line. I was grateful the surgeon did not stay long, for I needed to absorb and process what he had just told me.

After he left, I looked over at my roommate who had been following the conversation with unabashed curiosity—no, not with curiosity, but with human interest. I couldn't speak and neither did she; we just smiled at each other, both with tears streaming down our faces. She fully recognized the significance of what had just happened in the bed beside her. I was still feeling a lot of pain, but a huge pressure had been lifted from me.

I must have slept a little because, when I woke up, both Vincent and Pa were standing by my bed. Vincent, who does not like hospitals at all, looked acutely uncomfortable. I knew I looked very pale and was hooked up to an IV and still had the oxygen prongs in my nose. I was also not wearing my wig; instead, I had a stretch turban on my head. This was not what mothers should look like. I didn't really know it, but I now looked as ill as I was. That day in that hospital room, there was no pretending possible. I looked like a cancer patient! I did not have hair, I did not have color on my face, and I did not have much energy. But I did have a clear margin and I did have clean lymph nodes and I did have my breast! I told my son and my dad this life affirming news. Pa understood the significance of it immediately, but Vincent was too anxious by all that he saw to fully realize it.

He just wanted to get out of that hospital room. He looked like he wanted to be away from that place, strongly smelling of disinfectants, and away from the person in the bed who hardly resembled his mother. He could not wait to get out into the fresh air. At the same time he also did not want to leave. He wanted to reassure himself that his mom was really OK. I told both of them about the size of the tumor and that all the nodes taken were clear. I could see in Pa's face the relief I also felt. The two of them left shortly after that, so I could rest. A nurse came in to give me painkillers, and I fell peacefully into a healing sleep.

Later, another nurse woke me up asking me if I needed more painkillers. I did not need any, for which I was glad. I would not need painkillers again. I wanted to rid my body as soon as possible from the offensive substances. I was not being a martyr: If I had been in unbearable pain, I would most definitely have accepted the painkillers. There was pain, certainly, but it was bearable. I wanted to support the healing, and I felt that taking pain medication when I did not really need it was not supportive of my immune system. I had brought my vitamin supplements with me to the hospital. I used most of them in the hospital, except the Shark Cartilage because it constricts the blood vessels and this is not safe after surgery.

One night, while I was in a deep sleep, a nurse woke me up. Not to ask me, as many had previously, if I needed painkillers, but whether I used visualization to control the pain. I had not used that. To me it did not make sense to wake up a patient from a healing sleep to ask this question. Was she writing my answer in her report? Patient 589,898 did not want painkillers after surgery. I did not need painkillers; because the pain was bearable it was as simple as that. But it was probably not simple to them, because most people do ask for more painkillers, not less.

My roommate, who had walked with me a short distance on my road, only stayed one night. She was discharged the next day. After that, I was alone! No other patient came to stay in the bed next to me. I also did not see many nurses during the day. At night, I slept, so I did not know whether they came in then. Since I was mostly resting and sleeping, I had not realized that this was somewhat odd. I became aware of it when one nurse came in and asked me whether I had noticed that the nurses were not coming into my room.

"We are all scared," she said. "When someone about the same age most of us are comes in with breast cancer, we find it very difficult to come into your room."

I had been in hospitals before and knew that nurses are

in and out of your room most of the time. I had actually been enjoying the quiet, between visitors. It gave me lots of time to rest and focus on healing. So I had not minded not seeing the nurses. After all, if I needed them I could always ring the bell. They should probably have checked on me, because what if there had been complications and I had been unable to push the button for the bell? I was so thankful that had not happened.

I did have many visitors. Shirley, my other boss, was my first visitor the day after surgery. She brought me a beautiful guardian angel pin. Dan—my boss, friend, and one of my biggest supporters, had made soup and brought whole-wheat bagels. I could not find much on the menu, which suited my very strict self-imposed diet. Even the Heart Smart diet was filled with margarine, white bread, overcooked vegetables, and Jell-O with food coloring. I ordered and picked from the menu what I felt were the least unhealthy items, but I was glad for Dan's soup and bagels. I felt nurtured and taken care of by my visitors. They were also my link with the outside world, a world I wanted to return to quickly. The day after my surgery, a team of about 10-12 Medical students came in with the surgeon. The surgeon was very pleased with how quickly the surgical site was healing. With the team standing in the back, as if not wanting to be seen, stood the young doctor whose talk about stimulating your immune system I had been to during the early part of my journey. She did not participate in the interactions between students and teacher. My surgeon teaches at the faculty of Medicine. She appeared to be only there to observe. Why was she there? Was she a student? Was she a teacher? Was I part of her research? I don't know any of these answers, and I did not see her again.

After a few days, I was discharged and went home. I had an external tube drain in place, to prevent fluid and blood from accumulating under the skin. The drain continuously removed fluid from the surgery site into an external collection device. It gave me quite a bit of discomfort. I had very little mobility in my left arm. The drain was irritating the skin around it and had to be emptied manually every day. I would not ask Vincent to do this and so tried to do it myself. Irene, my rowing buddy, came for a visit and noticed that Vincent and I were barely managing. She was wondering why I was not assigned help from homecare.

She called the health nurse who came out and asked many questions. She asked me if Vincent knew how to cook, which he did not. She asked me if Vincent was in school full-time, which he was. She asked me how I was managing with the drain, and I showed her how difficult it was. She asked if there was anyone in the house who could help me with the drain. I explained that there was only Vincent and how tough all of this was on him and that seeing blood had always strongly affected him to the point that he even passed out from the sight of blood in the past. She asked me how I was managing normal household chores, but she could see that I was too weak to do much of anything myself. Vincent was mostly gone during the day and did his best to help as much as he could, but we needed more help.

She said I definitely qualified for homecare. She would phone it in. When she did, she called me back to let me know that she was not successful in securing homecare for us, because it should have been initiated by the hospital. Why had the hospital not ordered it? Or asked me if I had help or needed it? I was a single parent with a 14-year-old son. Irene phoned the hospital for answers, and she was told that I had seemed so capable.

When Irene told me this, I asked her who had decided that. There had hardly been anyone in my hospital room to see me. I had only received the bare minimum care. It had been difficult for me to bathe or take a shower, yet only once had there been someone in to assist me. I had to fend largely for myself because of the nurses' fears. I had shuffled to the fridge to get my soup and bagel. I had refused more pain medication. Had someone interpreted this as being very capable? Yes, normally, I am a very capable person, but I had just had major surgery and could barely move my left arm because of the large number of lymph nodes that had been removed. Because of the area where the nodes were taken, nerves and muscles were affected. I had a drain, which needed daily attending, a household to run, and only a 14-year-old son to help me. I needed help. But the help I was entitled to was not available for me.

Earlier in the hospital, while I was waiting for the surgery, the breast cancer nurse had come in to the waiting room to talk to me. She said that most of the information she would give me I had probably already received from my support visitor from *Reach to Recovery*. I told her that no one had contacted me from *Reach to Recovery*. She appeared a little taken aback when she heard that and asked if I wanted someone from *Reach to Recovery* to contact or visit me. I said "Yes." I explained to her that not only did I want it now, I would also have welcomed it when I was first diagnosed. Why had I not been contacted earlier by *Reach to Recovery*?

Did I look capable on paper, too? Or was it just another coincidence? Was it because I had initially refused traditional methods? Was it all part of having to travel this road alone? Will these questions ever be answered? I did receive a call after I came home from surgery from *Reach to Recovery*. A personable young woman came out to visit me. We had a very nice visit. I again questioned why I had not received a visit earlier. I was certainly not given the choice or asked the question, because no one had called me earlier. It was the same with the support for homecare. I was not asked if I needed help.

A little while later, at my first appointment with the oncologist after surgery, he had explained that usually they start radiation after a lumpectomy. But this time he did not tell me that is what I had to do. Instead he explained to me that this was customary, and then he asked me what I would like to do. When I heard him ask me a question instead of telling me what to do, I almost fell off my chair. Was this the same doctor who had so unkindly exclaimed, when I did not follow his recommendation, that he could not guarantee that my breast would be saved? Was this also the same doctor who had been so insensitive the day I came in for chemotherapy? Was this the same person who now asked me what I wanted to do? I answered him, honestly, that

I didn't know much about Radiation and I would like to speak with someone, so that I could gather information. He referred me to the head of Radiation, so I could meet with him and he would be able to give me information.

After I changed from a gown back into my own clothes, I opened the door and was getting ready to leave the hospital. When I came out of the examination room, I saw the oncologist standing by a desk talking with another doctor. When I started walking down the hall towards the stairs I heard someone loudly call out my name. I turned and saw that it was the oncologist shouting to me from where he was standing. Then he proceeded to point to the man standing next to him as he yelled at me, "This is the doctor you will see." It seemed quite out of character for this normally quite reserved doctor to call out to me across the hall. I suspect strongly that it was not so much for me to see who the head of Radiation was, as for that doctor to see who I was. It is of course possible that I am reading far too much into things. I could be wrong. However, this does not change the fact that my oncologist's actions were odd that day.

I did meet with the head of radiation. But after meeting with him and trying to get information from him I could not think of good reasons to have radiation. None of the information I received from him could convince me that having radiation was beneficial for me. According to the surgery report, the surgeon had found an encapsulated small tumor and there was a clear margin. It was a slow growing medullary cancer and the risk of it spreading was low. So why then would I subject myself to lowering my immune system through radiation? I wanted to strengthen my immune system, so that I could become increasingly healthy. The radiation specialist also told me that this would be localized radiation therapy. I did not think this was true and told him so; after all, my blood flowed through the localized area and so would become radiated. He did not answer me when I asked him to explain this to me.

There was an information session for people who had already given signed consent for Radiation treatment. I had not given consent, but asked if I could go to the information session anyway. I was told that I could not go to that information session, unless I gave written consent that I would take radiation treatment. Permission for me to attend the information session was denied! I was not allowed to go unless I gave signed consent. I did not feel I had enough information to go ahead and take radiation therapy.

So I left feeling that I could now concentrate on getting stronger and healing from the treatment. I felt secure in the knowledge that there had been a clear margin, and I wanted to leave the anxiety and stress behind me: I wanted to get on with my life and have as little as possible to do with the mainstream medical community—I wanted as much as possible to forget them.

Chapter Fifteen

Pressure from the Cancer Clinic

I was not yet aware of it, but I was being observed and I was being discussed. The tumor, which had been sent to the lab, was very much noticed and very much discussed. Something strange had occurred, something which defied explanation. When the journey had first begun earlier in the year, a biopsy had been performed and tissue had been taken. The results from that biopsy showed that the tumor consisted of aggressive ductal cancer cells. But something was highly unusual because the tumor, which had been removed in September during surgery, showed a different kind of cancer. What was found at that time was a low-grade medullary cancer. Something was very strange. It was most certainly not the same type of cancer. What was happening?

Not yet known to me, I would soon find out that discussions by the breast cancer team were taking place. The entire team examined both slides with the two different types of cancer cells on it. The team examined and discussed, and it was then decided by the cancer team that the findings from the surgery were not correct. I was not given any details about how they came to this conclusion, but I was told that the cells sent to the lab during and after surgery, which had shown a low grade medullary cancer was wrong. It was then further decided by the team that the cells taken from the first biopsy were the correct ones and that I had a highly aggressive ductal cancer. Based on this, they insisted that I needed more treatment.

It would have been very interesting to have been a fly on the wall during these discussions because the interesting facts remained: Two different types of cancer cells were found two different times. Because of this inconsistency, the team assumed that one had to be wrong. They decided that the last diagnosis, based on my surgery result, the one that had found the low-grade medullary cancer, was wrong. As a result of these findings, a letter was sent to my family doctor urging her to insist that I return to the cancer clinic and take more treatment—not just to finish the chemotherapy course, but to have the six weeks of radiation I had also refused.

After my meetings with the head of the Radiation Department and my check up visit with the oncologist, I had continued with my healthy eating regimen: taking supplements, praying, participating in both Psychosynthesis and immune-stimulating chiropractic treatments. I had another friend who had introduced me to a man who practiced therapeutic touch and had received two sessions from him. Sherron, from my office, is married to a Mormon bishop, and I had been to her house where he and two other men from the Mormon Church had prayed over me and asked for a blessing. My name had been added to numerous prayer lists from various churches, including Catholic, Mormon, Protestant, Evangelical, and Pentecostal. Not only Christian people were praying for me, but Muslim, Hindus, and Buddhists as well. I continued to have a wall of prayer around me.

I was healing well after the surgery and was beginning to feel strong again. I had not received the home care I was entitled to, but many people had brought food and helped clean my house: Their help gave me another boost and helped me feel nurtured and cared for. Accepting help was still not easy for me, and asking for it almost painful, but I was learning. There was, however, a minor setback in my learning; it happened only days after I returned home from the hospital. It had been my own stubborn doing.

When I had first returned home after surgery, a local grocery store had their monthly $1.49 day. Vincent and I always enjoyed going there because of the huge savings. We also needed many groceries items, so I decided that I was strong enough to go there, as long as Vincent was with me. Big mistake! By the time we had paid for the groceries, I was so exhausted that it was only through sheer mental will that I was able to make it back to the car. Concentrating on one painful step after another, all I could think about was, "If I can get into the car and sit down, I can drive myself home and then I can collapse on the couch."

I did not hear the carry-out girl ask me if I was all right, so intense was my concentration on trying to walk to the car. Vincent told me about it later when I was finally sitting in the driver's seat and after they had put the groceries in the car together.

He asked me if I had not heard the girl talk to me and why I had not answered when she asked whether I was all right.

"Why," I asked, "do I look sick?" He answered worriedly, "Mom, you look so pale, are you OK?" I told him that I was just a little tired, which was quite an understatement. Of course, I should not have pushed myself to the grocery store, because my body needed to heal, and I could have seriously set back my recovery. I was lucky that did not happen. So many people were available for help. All I had to do was ask. I had nothing to prove, so it was totally unnecessary that I had gone shopping, especially since I usually don't even like shopping.

I thought everything was going very well until the day when my family doctor's nurse called to ask me to come in and see my doctor. I had no idea what was happening. I also had a physiotherapy appointment in the same building to help me regain mobility in my arm. Thirty two lymph nodes had been removed. According to my family doctor, I had radical surgery without the loss of my breast. She had looked at both scars. There was one on my breast and another long one under my left armpit. She had said, "They were digging, yes: They were looking for cancer." They were the surgeon and his team, and they had not found it. All lymph nodes were clean!

But after the diagnostic team had looked and discussed my conflicting biopsy and surgery report, they had decided that the second diagnosis was wrong. Even the fact that no cancer was found in any of the 32 lymph nodes they had removed did not seem to make a difference. So, when I received a call from my doctor's office, I went there unsuspecting, still under the impression that all was well, and I was getting better and stronger every day. I was feeling optimistic and hopeful, but it became very apparent that my family doctor did not share my feelings. She was quite obviously scared the day I went to see her. She showed me a letter, which had been sent to her by the cancer team, and after reading that letter I, too, became very scared. I call this letter the fear letter and, after reading it, I told her I did not know what to do. She gave me a copy of the letter and asked me to please go back and finish the treatment recommended in it. The letter stated that I should return immediately and finish the three months of chemo I had started but had not finished in July, and then add to those six weeks of radiation to be taken after that.

What I did not know, then, was that there were also telephone conversations between the doctors of the cancer Clinic and my family doctor. She was told that if I did not return for and finish the treatment, I would not see the end of 1996 and I would be dead before the year was over. She was very scared for me. And after seeing her, I was now scared and confused, too. Even though I was recovering well from the surgery, I was still fragile physically. This affected my mental and emotional steadiness. Seeing my family doctor and being cautioned by her to return for the treatment only helped to make me feel more scared and confused. I had known what to do intuitively before the surgery; now, I was feeling very bewildered, scared, and lost.

I left my doctor's office not knowing where to turn or what to do. I still had to go to my physiotherapy appointment. I went upstairs to the physiotherapy department with a very heavy heart. I was taken behind a curtain where I sat on a cot and waited for the therapist. It was a young woman I had never seen before and would never see again. Again, the timing of seeing this young woman was significant because what she told me helped me to find the right answer for me. I was feeling so vulnerable that when she came in and asked me how I was, I burst into tears. The fear and confusion were erupting. It all came pouring out. I told her what had just happened downstairs at my family doctor's office and what my journey had been like prior to all this.

I also showed her the letter and told her I had been so sure before reading it that I was now fine. I had thought that the surgery had been a success and that I just needed to work on healing and getting stronger, that the worst was now behind me, and that I no longer needed to focus on the fight, but on the recovery instead. I also told her that reading the letter had changed all that. Now, I was not only very confused, but very scared. After the surgery, I had seen the pathology report. I had thought that all the cancer was removed and that the fight was almost over. But now, with this letter, I didn't know what to do, what to think, what to feel. I was very confused.

This young woman, the physiotherapist, did not advise me; she listened quietly with warm compassion, and when I was finished, she suggested that I find a calm spot inside myself. "That's where your answer is," she told me. She said that inside me I would find the answer about what I should do, I would discover and know with certainty what the right action would be for me to take.

Having been able to talk about it to someone who did not seem to be scared and who was not emotionally attached to me, but who could be an unbiased observer, had calmed me down, and had empowered me. I instinctively felt that what she had told me was affirmative and that I should find that quiet place inside myself and just be still, trusting that the answer would come. And over the next few days I did just that.

Meanwhile, my oncologist's nurse had also phoned me to make sure I was aware of the letter sent and to let me know how important it was that I come back a. s. a. p. to the cancer clinic to finish the recommended treatments. She asked me what I was going to do. I told her I was not sure, that I had to think about what I was going to do. She voiced her concern and told me not to take too much time.

The nurse asked whether it would help me if other patients were to phone me, ones who were of similar age to me with a similar diagnosis and who were receiving similar treatment as the one recommended to me. Since I was again trying to collect information and had not yet found what I was to do next, I said I would talk to other patients and that she could give other patients my phone number. Once more, she emphasized that I not take too long to decide, and she asked me for a commitment to let her know by the end of the week what my decision would be. I promised her I would do that.

Not long after that, a young woman phoned me. I think she was very kind by calling me. She must have strongly believed that she was helping me. And she did help me, but not in the way she, or the oncologist's nurse, had intended or expected. She explained the treatments she had undergone and was still undergoing. She also told me her story, and we ended up talking about ourselves. She owned a flower shop, was about my age, not married, and did not have children. Her boyfriend had broken up with her when she was first diagnosed with cancer. She had no hair from her chemo treatments, and she had gained a lot of weight, also from the chemo treatment. She sounded very depressed. In an unguarded moment she said sadly, "I am fat, bald and alone."

She had exposed her vulnerability to me, and I felt great sadness for her. She'd uttered those words with such deep despair that it made my heart ache. She explained to me that the treatment she was getting had left her sterile. She told me that she had always wanted children and, now, she would forever be unable to ever have any of her own. Since she knew I had made choices different from hers, she asked me what I had been doing instead of radiation and chemotherapy. I gave her a condensed version of all that I had been and was still doing. Somehow, she did not seem to hear that I had radically changed my eating habits, was taking supplements, drinking purifying teas, did not eat sugar or drink caffeine. She also did not appear to understand that I had a wall of prayer around me and was doing Psychosynthesis and receiving immune boosting treatments from my chiropractor. It appeared that she only heard that I had given up the fat in my diet. "Oh," she said, "I could never give up fat." I was taken aback by her reaction. A part of me wanted to reply to her, "Yes, but you did give up having children."

But, I couldn't say that to her—that would be so cruel, so insensitive: She already sounded so sad and depressed. She was trying to help me decide. She had called me wanting to assist me in my decision, thinking that the treatment she had chosen would save our lives. She did help me decide but it was to not go ahead and have more treatment. My conversation with her helped confirm for me and make it very clear to me that I would NOT have more treatment. I resolutely decided that I would continue the immune boosting alternative non-invasive treatments I was currently giving myself. But I was not yet at the point where I could voice it out loud, so I did not tell her how speaking with her had helped me make a decision. Besides, what purpose would that have served? She believed in the choice she had made and seemed to be firmly supporting it. Less than two years later, by chance, I read her obituary. She had lost her fight.

Chapter Sixteen

The Dress!

Before my visit with my family doctor, and before the arrival of The Fear Letter, I had said to Jenni, "Let's go and get party dresses." I wanted to celebrate life, and to show I was doing that, I wanted a party dress! In my adult life, I had never had much money to speak of. I had lived a very frugal life for many years, for there was never much money. Nevertheless, my life was rich in many other ways. However, owning a party dress just did not fit into the frugal life style I was leading. I owned pretty clothes, and certainly had dresses that I wore to parties, but a dress which could only be worn to one event, a party, I did not own. Now I not only wanted such a dress, I needed to own a dress like that. And I knew just what kind of dress it had to be. It had to be the kind of dress that when you look at it, you have no doubt it was a party dress! I also did not want to buy it On Sale. I had always bought anything I wanted On Sale. This time, because of the symbolic significance, I wanted to buy it by paying Full Price! I was worth it!

So Jenni and I set out to buy ourselves party dresses. I didn't know what it would look like, but I knew that I would recognize it when I saw it. It was close enough to Christmas and New Years that the holiday party dresses were already in the stores. We had planned to take all afternoon for our party dress shopping adventure. I do not like shopping, so what happened next was pure magic.

We entered the first store, and I walked straight to a rack filled with party dresses. Somehow I did not even see any of the other dresses—I saw only one! I took it off the rack. I held it up and showed it to Jenni. Seeing it on the hanger does not do it justice, yet at that moment I fell in love with that dress. I was seeing what others could not see.

Jenni looked at the size; it was a size 12. "You are not a size 12," she said. She was right: I had been size 16-18, months earlier. "Oh, I know," I said, "but I want to try this dress on anyway, just for fun, I won't do up the zipper; I just want to try it on." And so, after Jenni also found a few dresses, we went into the change rooms. I had only taken The Dress in with me. I had not even looked at other dresses.

In the change room, I carefully put on the dress. I slid it over my head and oh, so carefully, moved it over my hips. Amazingly, so far, it fit! But I had not yet done up the zipper. I was fully expecting not to be able to pull it up, let alone all the way. But as I tried, it slid higher and higher, until it zipped all the way to the top. I had hardly breathed during this process. I had also not looked at myself in the mirror, yet. I expected that I would probably look like a stuffed sausage in this pretty dress. Just because I could zip up the zipper all the way to the top did not mean the dress fit. But in my mind's eye, I looked fabulous and I felt great in my chosen party dress. I wanted to stay with my imaginary look as long as possible. But I heard Jenni's voice asking me from her change booth whether the dress fit. There was no mirror inside my little cubby; in order for me to see what I looked like, I had to come out.

I walked out of the change room and, at that moment, everyone stopped what they were doing and turned to look at me. I still did not know what they were seeing. I looked to find a mirror and when I did, I finally saw what they all saw. There in the mirror was the image of a pretty woman in a stunning dress, and the dress fit as if it was made for her. And that woman was me! I twirled and pranced; I looked over my shoulder into the mirror. The dress looked so gorgeous, and I felt so alive, so beautiful. I did not want to take off that dress, ever.

"This is the dress!" I exclaimed to Jenni. She nodded; she, too, could see that it was. Reluctantly, I finally took it off. Afterwards, some of the women trying on dresses told me that they had seen it on the rack but had not realized how stunning it would look on someone. Me! It looked stunning on me!

The dress is black silk, covered in sparkling jet beads. It is a very heavy dress and very impractical. But party dresses are not meant to be practical. It is tailored, with a scooped, round neckline (both in the front and in the back); short, sculpted sleeves; and three skirts (also covered with beads) cascading down to just above my knees. It looks a little like a flapper dress, but it is shorter. It is the kind of dress you can wear to opening night at the opera or wear dancing. I not only found it, but I was able to buy my party dress! I had wanted to pay full price, but I had not realized how much party dresses actually cost. Yet, somehow, I had enough money to pay for this dress. It was priced under $60, which is quite unbelievable. I feel that this dress was just waiting for me to find it.

It was also this dress that helped me to decide what to do next in my fight against cancer. It was early Friday afternoon; the time given to me before I had to decide what to do next was almost up. I had promised the oncologist's nurse that I would give her my decision that day. I still had not made a definite choice, even though I was close to knowing what I would do next. I went to my closet and I don't know why, but I picked up The Dress from the closet. I held it up in front of me, to look at its beauty, its style. To me, this dress symbolized LIFE. And at that moment, holding that dress, I knew with clear certainty what was right for me. I would choose life. I chose the dress, and I would also choose not to have any more treatment. I would phone the nurse and tell her my final decision.

But I didn't have to, because just then, the phone rang. I answered it, and I was not at all surprised to discover that it was the nurse. Holding the dress in one hand, and the phone in the other, and with my eyes fixed on my dress, I told the nurse, my voice clear and strong, "I have decided not to have any more treatment: I am of sound body and mind, and you have given me all the information possible." I then continued, "I have spoken with the other cancer patient, and having all this knowledge, I am choosing not to have any more treatment."

The nurse could probably hear the seriousness of what I had just said in my voice. My voice, which was now strong and full of conviction, did not waver. I'm not sure whether she realized that nothing she would say at this time could or would change my mind, but she did not even try. She acknowledged that she had heard me, and we ended the conversation.

I was finally not only able to listen to my own voice, but I was now acting on it as well. I looked at the dress and felt grounded and strong. I had chosen LIFE. And this choice would give me life, of that I was now very certain.

But I wanted a guarantee, so I asked God for a guarantee. This was the answer I received. Later that day Vincent and I drove to the store. It was early evening, but since it was December, it was already very dark. We were in the car on our way out of the parking lot, when I saw a truck driving at least 50 km, speeding straight towards us. He was not just heading towards us; he was aimed straight towards the driver's side, my side. He was driving at high speed and was most certainly going to hit the driver's side, where I was sitting. His speed was so fast that he would certainly kill me and maybe my son, too, on impact.

At that moment, I saw my life flash before me and thought, somewhat surprised, "How can this be, but I'm going to be hit by a truck and die in my car!" Again, time played one of its tricks. Milliseconds became drawn-out minutes. Time seemed suspended. The truck was still approaching, very fast. It is hard to realize that everything took place in minuscule amounts of time. The speeding truck passed a stop sign. It should have stopped him. He ignored it and continued flying through it without even slowing down. Was he drunk? I tried to get out of the way, but knew I would not have enough time to do so. I was moving too slowly to be gone by the time he reached us.

And then, just as the truck was about to hit us, it was as if two giant hands moved us just enough so the truck only barely touched the front corner of my car. It didn't even feel like we had hit each other, but I knew the two vehicles had touched each other. He came to a squealing stop. I had already stopped. I looked at the shaken driver who was still inside his truck. We both got out of our vehicles. His first words were, "I didn't see you!" Well, that had been obvious. He looked at the front of my car and said, "Well, it doesn't look like any damage, I'll just move on." It was a dark parking lot, and I knew we could not see everything clearly, and I told him that. I insisted on taking his insurance information anyway, which he appeared reluctant to give: If he did not see any damage, he may have thought that it was totally unnecessary. But he complied and we shared insurance information, then we both went on our respective ways. It turned out there was some minor damage to my car, and his insurance would pay for it.

But something else had happened: I had received my answer from God. The answer was, "You don't get a guarantee about life, because nobody does, you could be hit by a truck!"

To make sure I really got the message, exactly a week later, at around the same time, Vincent and I were hit by a truck again. We were getting ready to leave another parking lot and were stopped in front of the stop sign, when behind us another truck was getting ready to stop. He hit a patch of ice and was unable to stop in time before he hit our car. This time the shaken up driver was very apologetic: He had seen us, and he had tried to stop, but was unable to do so. He gave us his insurance information without me having to ask for it. This time there was no damage. But the message was the same: "You do not get a guarantee, life does not come with guarantees, and you could be hit by a truck!" At that point in my discussions with God, I said, "OK, OK, I got it; please do not send any more trucks!" And no other trucks were sent to hit us.

I did not have any contact with Medical Personnel during the remaining part of 1996. I was not, as the oncologist, radiologist and surgeon had predicted, dying! I was taking my party dress dancing. I had told all my friends I needed a date for my dress because I wanted to take my dress dancing. Everyone, including myself, was looking for a date for me and my dress. It would be Dan and his wife Ann, who would find a date for me and The Dress. I remember we went out for a wonderful Italian dinner, that my date was nice and that he could dance, but I don't remember the man's name.

When we walked into the dancehall, the first person I saw was a member of the small live band, the singer, and I knew him! As fate would have it, his name was Joy! I know it was a sign. He greeted me warmly, and his face and voice showed admiration for the way I looked in my party dress. The band began to play, and when I walked onto the dance floor, Joy spoke into the microphone dedicating the first song they played to me. Life was good! Although my date was a good dancer, my friend and supporter Dan is a fabulous dancer. During one of my dances with him, Joy again spoke into the microphone to address me directly by saying, during an instrumental solo, "You're looking good Margreet!" I could not have imagined a more perfect night for my dress, and I was in it, enjoying life! It was a perfect celebration for the finished fight. In 1996, instead of dying, I was busy living and would continue to have wonderful healing experiences full of personal growth and Joy! So I ended that long, difficult year, 1996, dancing!

Chapter Seventeen

1997: More healing

LYMPHEDEMA: 1998

The next year, 1997, I went back to Holland to visit Ieke. It had been 21 years since I had last been to my birth country. Ieke had given me a wonderful gift. She told me, when she had visited in June of 1996, during our visit in my little back yard, that anytime I wanted to come to Holland, she would send me a ticket and I could stay with her. She pampered me greatly during this visit. Every morning, she spoiled me with freshly squeezed orange juice and breakfast in bed. Even though I could have taken this journey overseas in between my treatments, I had decided to wait until the fight was over. The trip to the place where I was born and had spent the first 16 years of my life was also part of my healing. Ieke and I visited the house I grew up in and I was able to release more ghosts. My best friend from high school and I went to visit my high school sweetheart, and I could finally release him, too. Although I came back from Holland with a Dutch bike, I was much lighter because of what I had been able to lay to rest, and finally leave behind.

That year, the year after the surgery, 1997 I also developed lymphedema. Lymphedema is a common chronic condition where excess fluid, called lymph, collects in the tissues and causes swelling in them. Lymphedema can happen as a result of surgery after lymph vessels and lymph nodes are surgically removed. When these vessels or nodes are gone, it can interrupt the normal drainage of the lymphatic fluid. Lymphedema is usually not life threatening; however, the swelling does not necessarily or entirely go away after the onset of lymphedema. I now have a swollen left hand and arm; sometimes it is worse than others, but the swelling never goes away. I manage it with a compression sleeve and glove. My lymphedema occurred after I did some gardening.

I was on a plant rescue mission. Not very far from where Vincent and I lived, there were two trailer courts. Because of Real Estate value at this location, the sites were sold and all trailers had to be moved. The trailer court had been there for more than 20 years, and many people had lovely little gardens with mature perennial plants. I knew that they would be plowed under to make room for development. It saddened me to think of all these plants that had been growing there for years. So I convinced Jenni one evening to go with me to look at the plants. We had to duck under some wire surrounding the now deserted area. We were amazed at the many beautiful mature plants, shrubs, and trees that would soon no longer exist. I could not let them be killed. I wanted to rescue all of them, but my garden was not big enough for all.

While Jennie and I were strolling together in the twilight around the deserted trailer court, we witnessed a magic moment. As the sun set, there sprung, suddenly before us, a beautiful white rabbit. He was not afraid, and the three of us enjoyed a moment together in time. Just as unexpectedly as he had appeared, he disappeared. And I, always looking for a sign, interpreted this as a signal that what I was doing was supported by the Universe.

So the next day, armed with a shovel, plastic bags, and garden fork, I set out on my rescue mission. I had given some thought to which plants I would reclaim. One I really wanted was Hops. I also chose some Lilies and an Alberta Rose. I had looked around the abandoned trailer court and knew exactly where they were. I drove to them and opened the trunk of my car. I covered it with plastic and started to dig. I filled my entire trunk with plant treasures. When my trunk was full, I drove home and dug holes in my own backyard where I planted the salvaged plants. It wasn't until I was finished that I noticed how tight the skin of my left hand felt. When I looked at it, I noticed that it was quite swollen. Immediately, I realized what the swelling meant. What I did not realize, then, was that it would be something that would remain with me, always, to more or lesser degrees: My hand and arm were swollen from lymphedema.

In 1998, two years and a day since my chemo treatment on July 17, 1998, I made an appointment with my family doctor. I had not seen her in, maybe, a year. She was excited to see me, as I was to see her. We were in the examination room, where I was sitting in the chair and she on the examination table. She smiled, but tears glistened in her eyes as she said, "So here you are!" And then she repeated it and said it again. I smiled back at her and said, "Yes, here I am." Then she told me that she considered me her miracle patient and proceeded to tell me why. That day she told me of the many frightening phone calls she had received from the cancer clinic. She asked me if I had realized that the people at the cancer Clinic had not thought that I would survive the year, that they believed I would not live to see 1997. Their diagnosis of the cancer had been that it was so aggressive, and that since I did not accept the treatments they offered, I would surely be dead by the end of the year. I was thankful that she had not shared this with me in 1996.

"And so here you are," she said again.

I smiled back at her and nodded, "yes, here I am."

We now both had tears in our eyes. To let that knowledge sink in, we remained silent for a few moments.

Then we began to talk, once more, about what a local breast cancer specialist had said—how three women could be identical in their diagnosis, age, everything, but one will have all the treatment and die; the next will also have all the recommended treatments and live, but have a recurrence; and the third woman, her cancer will never reoccur. He had said in his talk that what medical people are overlooking is the host. I agreed with her, and told her that people have talked to me, and asked me to talk to their loved ones who are diagnosed with cancer about what I did to save my life so they could duplicate it and by doing this, thereby save their lives. I explained to her that I answer them that I cannot do that because I feel the most important thing I did was believe in what I was doing and am still doing, with a deep knowledge it was the right thing for me: If a person believes in conventional treatments, I cannot and will not take that belief away from her/him. While talking with my doctor, I told her I didn't even really remember everything I took, ate, or drank, that year, in 1996. I said I know all of that contributed to my healing but, more importantly, it was that I mostly believed so passionately in what I was doing in spite of a lot of intrusive doubts to challenge me, as doubt (mine and others') had very much been a part of my journey.

Chapter Eighteen

Two Diagnoses?

But what had happened to me? And why were two very different types of cancer found? Or were there? I discussed this with my chiropractor.

"You've explained to me that cancer is a mutant cell; is it possible, then, that this cancer mutated into a different cancer? After all, we are only scratching the surface of what our bodies are capable of. What if, because of all the different things I was doing, the original cancer (a highly aggressive fast growing ductal cancer discovered in my first biopsy) mutated, changing into a slow-growing medullary cancer, the cancer that was found when I had my surgery?"

He said that he thought it was possible. Meanwhile, the team at the cancer clinic was still convinced that it was ductal cancer.

And then, one day, in 1999, I went to see my family doctor for a minor medical concern. After we greeted each other, she said excitedly with a hint of amusement, "I have to show you something." She turned the computer screen on and showed me the latest letter sent to her from the cancer clinic. It was about me!

She said, "Look what it says." And there on the monitor, in plain sight, was what appeared to be a typical letter written from one doctor to another—except that, off handedly, it said I had been treated for medullary cancer.

"What is this?" I asked her.

"Well, obviously, they've changed their minds," she said. "It is because they can not explain what happened to you. Here you are, not only alive, three years later, but very healthy, with no sign of cancer."

She then said, "You know that I believe that a miracle happened, but most of the doctors at the hospital are looking at things from a scientific point of view only, so they have to explain it scientifically. The only way to do that is to change your diagnosis from aggressive ductal to the slow growing medullary, so that it all makes sense to them again, based on a scientific theory."

Then she asked me to come out of the room with her. She said, "I want to introduce you to someone."

She had a young medical student working with her that day. Together, we walked to the young woman and my family doctor said to her, "I want you to meet my miracle patient: This is Margreet Jansen van Doorn." The medical student seemed puzzled but I know that later my doctor would tell her the story of what happened in 1996 and, consequently, since then. She could see how healthy I looked, and my doctor would tell her how healthy I am.

I was curious to hear what my surgeon thought about the recent change of diagnosis. He had previously impressed me with his honesty. So I made an appointment to see him. He seemed pleased to see me, but he also said, in a tone which seemed somewhat accusatory, "It's been awhile since your last visit."

"Not that long," I replied. He looked at my chart to see how long it had been, and he was right: It had been a long time, a year and a half to be precise. Most people see their surgeon every 4-6 months. Well, I had been busy with life, and time had moved quickly. But I had come with a question and I wanted to hear his answer, his view on the situation. So I asked him: "What's up with this latest diagnosis? Why has it been changed again to medullary cancer?"

I expected an honest response, because he had always been

straightforward with me in the past. But his eyes, which had always made open contact, shifted to a point behind me. What was going on? Why did he not make direct eye contact with me? His answer was also vague. He spoke in typically obscure doctor language. But that was not how he had ever spoken to me previously. He had always been direct, honest and made strong eye contact. His choice of language had been clear and easy to understand. Not so today. If his face were not the same, I would have thought that he was a different doctor. His vague answers, as he continued to look somewhere to the side of me, had to do with how medullary cancer can mimic other types of cancer. He also said that I still had to be careful, but that I was basically O. K.

Well, I knew that. I knew I was O.K. But why was he so evasive with me that day? Why did his answers seem so vague? I tried to ask another question, hoping to access the honest man who had impressed me earlier. I asked him the same question I had asked Dr. Jones earlier, "Is it not possible that both diagnoses were correct, but that because of everything I did the aggressive ductal cancer had mutated into a slow growing medullary cancer?"

Still not making direct eye contact, he said, "Probably not." But I had to keep trying, so I continued and said, "You are the researcher; please keep an open mind—is it not possible that a mutant cell can mutate into something else?"

And then I finally saw a glimpse of the earlier honesty I so admired. Almost reluctantly he said, "I've never heard of it."

I tried again: "All I ask," I implored, "is that you keep an open mind and consider that possibility."

He didn't respond. And I knew that for whatever his reasons were, an honest conversation between two people was not possible that day. He spoke to me like a doctor to a patient and sadly and very disappointedly, I knew I would not return to him again. How could I trust him when I did not feel that he was telling me the entire truth? If I could not believe everything he said, how could I believe anything he said? I believe he was not truthful with me, that day.

Feeling disappointed, I left his office.

But I felt a vague gnawing inside my head. I felt I was overlooking something. Was he right? Had the medullary cancer mimicked the aggressive ductal cancer? How was that possible? Had it been slow growing non-aggressive all along, as they claimed? I walked to my car. I never park in the hospital parking lot, so it was a fair distance to my car. When I got close to my car, I suddenly knew what the gnawing thought was. It could not be true that it had been a slow growing medullary cancer from the beginning.

The facts are clear. In March of 1996, on my birthday, I had a full physical exam performed by my family doctor. It included a breast examination. She had not found anything suspicious in either of my breasts. One month later, in April of 1996, I found a lump the size of a dove egg. Then in July of 1996, the lump had grown to 3 x 4 inches (7 x 10 cm), and a second lump of 1 ½" (4 cm) was found under my left armpit in the lymph nodes. That was not a slow growing cancer; that was an aggressive, fast growing cancer. Whichever way you looked at it, in July of 1996, I had stage three cancer.

And I felt sad. Why could my surgeon not have given me honesty? Why could he not have talked to me like an equal, like the intelligent woman I knew I was?

He sent a superficial letter to my family doctor about how pleasant it had been to see me again. Another vagueness, "Pleasant," another generic word. It only added to my disappointment. Later, I had a chance to read the letters sent to my family doctor, written by the doctors at the cancer clinic. In one, I read that one of the doctors felt that this cancer behaved very aggressively. It was exactly what I had concluded after my visit to the surgeon, and I felt that my deductions were validated.

Later that year I auditioned for the play *Steel Magnolias* and did get the part of Truvy, the part that in the movie is played by Dolly Parton. It is a wonderful part, and I had to play her as both flamboyant and sexy. I had not realized that the entire cancer experience had left me with more than just physical scars. My scars are not as big as some, and I have not lost my breast, but I did lose a part of my breast and I have a perpetually swollen hand and arm. Playing flamboyant, feminine, sexy Truvy was important in reclaiming that part of me, healing my psyche after the battle.

I needed a publicity photo for the play. So I made an appointment with a photographer. He took some beautiful black and white photos, but when he offered to take some with me wearing just a robe around me, showing off my bare shoulders, I panicked. I didn't know what to say; it became apparent to me, then, that all was not well in my relationship with my body. Showing off skin, as he suggested, filled me with fear. I do believe this is a psychological side effect of battling breast cancer. Our breasts, in our society, are viewed so much as a part of our sexuality. One of my breasts had what looked like an ice-cream scoop dent missing from it covered by a large scar and I had another large scar under my arm. Both added to not feeling great about nudity and my sexuality. But playing Truvy helped.

When I had auditioned for the play, three parts were still not cast. I knew the movie well, because it is one of my favorites. The three parts were Quiser, played in the movie by Shirley Maclaine; M'Lynn, played in the movie by Sally Fields; and the part of Truvy. I felt I could play Quiser and M'Lynn well. I did not think I was the type of person who could play Truvy, but the director felt differently, because she saw that inside me, hidden, was Truvy. I needed flamboyant clothes and high-heeled shoes for the play. I did not have far to look for them. In my closet, I had a collection of colored high-heeled shoes and flamboyant clothes. I found Truvy's wardrobe in my own closet, just waiting to be dusted off and reclaimed. It was OK to look and feel like a woman again. The play was a huge success and was sold out for almost all performances.

Chapter Nineteen

Dragon Boat Team

SISTERSHIP 2

Later that year, 1999, after I had been for my 6 month check up, the same nurse who had earlier tried to get me to take more treatment told me about a dragon boat team for women living with breast cancer. In the local newspaper, I had read an article about it a year earlier. I had read that a team had been formed consisting of only women who lived with breast cancer; I had also read that the boat was full. So when she told me about it and asked me if I were interested I answered that I thought the boat was full.

"Yes," she said, "but they are forming a second boat, are you interested in joining?" I told her that I was, and so she gave me the information. That afternoon, I phoned, and even though that boat too was almost full, I did get a spot. The name of the dragon boat team is Sistership. For two years, I was a member of a dragon boat team for women who live with breast cancer. It was long enough to appear in a special calendar.

This 2001 calendar, made in 2000, was also very important to me. It was a calendar where all of us were tastefully unclothed. I, who had panicked at the suggestion to have my picture taken that showed my shoulders bare, was to be in a calendar, for all to see, standing at the edge of a river, wearing nothing else but a mosquito net.

It was another healing experience. I was reclaiming my

sensuality, sexuality and not afraid to show that having battled breast cancer does not mean that you are no longer attractive as a woman. I feel like the woman in the ad who is told, "You've come a long way baby." I surely have come a long way.

Being in a dragon boat race is really very exciting. I remember it now like it is happening this very moment.

We have just lined up and are in position, waiting for the signal. The crowd is watching us, but we don't look at them; we are all waiting for the start signal.

"Paddles up," and there it is—we are off.

Our paddles are down, and we push and pull them through the water. The boat surges forward. We have started the race. The drum's beat is pushing us to move faster. The crowd yells and cheers, but we can't hear them: All we hear is the beat of the drum, like a heart beat. The person directly in front of us determines our pace. That is the only person I can see. My friend Joyce sits next to me but I don't look at her.

I don't know how fast we are going. The water is splashing over me from different directions. I'm getting very wet. It's like rain, but the rain, which has threatened all day, is not there. It seems that just for our race, the sun has come out and is now shining on us. The day has just turned from dark and cloudy to sunny and bright. We would see it if we took the time to look. But we are too busy to be aware of the sun shining on us; we are pushing ourselves hard to get to the finish line.

This is more than a race for all of us—this has become symbolic of our struggle. Some of us are athletes; many of us are not. Some of us were even couch potatoes before we joined the team. But today, we are all here. We are all paddling as a team.

We move the paddles to lift and pull. Our breaths are getting ragged: It has only been one minute we have been paddling hard and, yet, we are being pushed by the drum to paddle harder. The drum's unrelenting beat drives us on, reminds us to keep going, to reach deeper inside ourselves, to reach the finish line, not to stop!

Ginny, who has just had reconstructive surgery, is too weak to paddle. But she beats the drum. It is the first time she has ever drummed because we did not have a drum prior to this day, yet she is drumming as if her life depends on it. We, too, are all paddling as if our lives depend on it, and in a way it does: this race is so symbolic of the greater race all of us have been running—the race for our lives. We are Sistership, and membership to this team does not come cheap. You have to have faced breast cancer to get into this boat.

The crowd cheers. Some people in the crowd cannot cheer. All they can do is look at us, and cheer in their hearts, with tears streaming down on their faces. But we can't see their tears or hear their voices; we only hear the insistent sound of our drum and sporadic sounds from the drums of the seven other dragon boats beside us.

Dragon Boats, Oriental fighting vessels which were traditionally used in Chinese wars, are for us, in this boat, a symbol of another fight: Our fight against breast cancer.

We hear the sound of the referee, "Boat number 5, stay in your lane." We know this is our boat, and we feel that we are not following a straight path, our boat is swerving. Freddie, who is steering us, is not very strong in her arms because of surgery, but she is trying valiantly to get us back into our lane. We should have been disqualified, because we have veered into another lane, but we are the crowd favorite and the referee knows it; any other boat would probably have been disqualified. Freddie manages to steer us straight again, but we have fallen behind. Ginny continues to pound on the drum.

We're all getting exhausted. Our bodies have endured so much in the past and, yet, we all push ourselves to our limits; we reach into our cores and find more strength—we will finish the race. In the crowd, watching us, are our fathers and mothers, our sons and daughters, our husbands, our lovers, our sisters and brothers, our friends. They all watch and cheer us on. They have felt so helpless before, when they could only watch us fight breast cancer; now they see we are not only alive, but that we are paddling a very stressful race, with the bodies that earlier had seemingly betrayed us; we keep going forward, and they keep watching us.

One final burst of energy, and we have finished the race. The crowd goes wild. We have come in sixth, but we were the ones they were waiting for to finish and we have done it. Sweat is pouring down our faces, we are all soaked, but we are so exhilarated! We have finished the race! We paddle back to the shore behind the other dragon boats, which have reached the finish line before us. We become aware just how exhausted we are. The boat is closer to shore and, now, we also become aware of the cheering and yelling of the crowd. Freddie steers us to the dock.

Ginny has stopped drumming. We still have one more thing to do before we get out of the boat. We all reach to the bottom where we have kept carnations, and we gently float them away on the water. These flowers are for all the sisters who cannot be a part of our team, the women who did not finish the race and whose lives have ended. Now the wetness from the water and sweat on our faces is mixed with tears. We get out of the boat and lift our paddles high in a final salute to the sky. To life, to a race completed! In unison we exclaim, "Yesssssss!!!!!!"

Epilogue

Life Goes On

On May 17, 2002, I was at the cancer Clinic in the morning for my annual check up, and on that day I was released from the cancer clinic! That day the doctor I had been seeing for the past few years told me that they were going to set me loose. My mammogram had come back normal, and I no longer had to return to the cancer clinic for check ups. When she told me this, I started to cry, and I cried walking out of there and all the way home. Not tears of sadness. Tears of relief. Tears of gratitude. Tears for all the other people who did not walk out. But I did walk out of that place with my head held high and in great health. The doctor was taken aback when I started to cry. She didn't know me, so she would not, could not understand why I was crying. She tried interpreting it from her point of reference, thinking that I needed the security of the clinic and that I was not ready to fly out yet.

She could not have been more wrong. Going there has not been a place of security for me, at all, or a place of comfort as the previous recollections has shown: It had been quite the opposite. I could not even begin to explain that to her. My dealings with her have been good, kind, and nice, nothing grating, nothing ordinary, quite neutral. Her bedside manner is gentle and kind, even with a touch of warmth. But she had not been there when I refused conventional treatment, when I began the journey six years earlier, against the advice of the mainstream medical community. In this story, she would be characterized as more of a fringe player, which is why I did not even try to explain to her what my tears were for. The tears were also for the struggle I had faced and overcome, for the unknown road I had chosen to walk six years ago. The tears were for the phone calls to my family doctor to pressure her by telling her that her patient, me, would not see the end of 1996 if I did not return to finish the treatment. I did not go back for the treatment and, yet, that day, very healthy, with no sign of cancer, I was getting released from the cancer Clinic. For all those things, I cried.

And now it is the summer of 2005! I'm sitting in another wonderful backyard oasis garden retreat. It is not the same one as 1996, but just as wonderful. This garden is in Okotoks, Alberta, where I moved in 2002. Five years ago in 2000, I met a wonderful handsome kind man, named Paul. We married in August of 2002 and moved to this Bed and Breakfast community south of Calgary. My life is amazing—it is full and blessed! My life is a continuing adventure. My job as parent educator is highly rewarding.

Two amazing little boys came into my life as a special gift. In 2000, they lived with Vincent and me for seven months before they were adopted by a very special family. I know I made a difference in their lives. If the cancer had won, I could not have done this. But the cancer did not win. I did and in my role as a parent educator/parenting coach, I continue to empower parents to encourage them to be the best teachers for their children. My life is worthwhile. Life is valuable and treasured.

My promise to myself is that I will not try to find the dark cloud behind the silver lining. Because I have for so long lived in the dark, where I had to find the silver lining, it is as if now that I am in the silver cloud looking for the dark lining. I will promise myself that I will not do that. I accept that. Life is Great! Life is a gift! Life is a miracle! Life is amazing! Life is joyful! Life is incredible! My life is awesome!

And so, even though death walks beside us everyday, life also walks beside us everyday, and it is up to us to decide and choose which partner we will accept. We can wait until death taps us on the shoulder to remind us that it is there before we start living, or we can start living right now. The choice is ours as long as we listen to our own drum to give us the beat, and we can start dancing!

And so here ends this part of my story. It is only a portion of my life. It impacted my life and gave me valuable lessons, but it remains only a portion, a chapter in the book of my life. And my story, the book of my life, will continue outside the pages of this book. New adventures will be found, other dragons will be faced and slain, there will be laughter, and there will be tears. There will be ups and downs. So it is.

NOTES

THE POWER OF HUMOR

"The art of medicine consists of keeping the patient amused while nature heals the disease." (Voltaire).

Humor has always been an important part of my life and it was no different during my experience with breast cancer. Long ago, Voltaire certainly understood that humor and laughter are good for your health. I always make sure humor is in my life, but it was even more important during my encounter with cancer. Of course, it is not easy to have a sense of humor when you need it the most—on the tough days. Yet, every year, there is more evidence to support that our emotions, moods, thoughts and belief system have a strong effect on our body's health and immune system. You've probably noticed yourself that you feel better after a good laugh. Our body's immune system is supported by love, hope, optimism, caring, intimacy, joy, laughter, and humor, and reacts negatively to hate, hopelessness, pessimism, indifference, anxiety, depression, loneliness, etc.

It is through the feelings we experience—or more accurately, through the neurochemical changes that come with these emotions--that our mind gets the power to influence whether we get sick or stay well.

Complex molecules called neuropeptides are found in our entire body, including the brain and immune system. These neuropeptides are how all cells in our body communicate with each other. This includes brain-to-brain messages, brain-to-body messages, body-to-body messages, and body-to-brain messages.

Individual cells, including brain cells, immune cells, and other body cells, have receptor sites that receive neuropeptides. The kinds of neuropeptides available to cells are changing constantly, based on our emotions throughout the day. The exact combinations of neuropeptides released during different emotional states have not yet been determined. But it is obvious that having more humor and laughter in our life helps make sure that these chemical messages are working for us, not against us.

Our daily mood or frame of mind gives us a powerful boost to our health. Our sense of humor is one of the most incredible tools we have to make sure our daily mood and emotional state support good health.

Humor helps us to relax muscles, reduce stress hormones, enhance our immune system, and reduce our pain.

THE POWER OF PRAYER

I was surrounded by a wall of Prayer. I found some intriguing information on the power of prayer and having a wall of prayer around me. I know that it has made a difference in my life and, interestingly, enough studies are being conducted that are beginning to support what I intuitively know. And just because a measuring instrument has not been invented or discovered yet does not mean that something is not real or does not exist. So, for your information, I have added the following on the power of prayer and being surrounded by a wall of prayer.

A study of cardiac patients was conducted at St. Luke's Hospital in Kansas City, Missouri. This study was published in the October 25, 1999 issue of the Archives of Internal Medicine. It concluded that a type of prayer—known as intercessory prayer—may, indeed, make a difference. Intercessory prayer is praying for strangers without their knowledge. The cardiac researcher William Harris, Ph. D who headed the study said, "Prayer may be an effective adjunct to standard medical care."

174

A group of Christian volunteers were praying for patients and were only given their first names. The patients were not told they were in a study, and the praying volunteers never visited the hospital. They were given instructions to pray for the patients daily, "for a speedy recovery with no complications." Dr. Harris used a long list of events that could happen to cardiac patients such as chest infections, pneumonia, and death. Dr. Harris' conclusion was that the group receiving the prayers did 11 percent better than the group that did not. This number is considered statistically significant. Dr. Harris said that his study supports the evidence that prayer works: "To me, it almost argues for another intelligence to have to redirect this very vague information."

THE POWER OF SUPPORT

I had a powerful team supporting me. The following gives you some information on the importance of a solid support system. People who have support of caring family and friends usually deal better with illness and are less likely to become depressed. They are also more independent, recover faster from illness, have lower blood pressure, and live longer.

Most of us know this from our own lives. Personally I usually felt better after sharing a cup of herbal tea with a friend, or after a phone call from someone who cares about me. Another benefit of being around people is that they can help take our mind off our illness.

When we are ill, relationships can be difficult because our friends and family may want more of our time and energy than we can give. I found it helped to teach them about my situation.

Talking about feelings and thoughts is often hard even in the best of times. When we are faced with a serious illness, it gets even harder. It's often easier to withdraw or say as little as possible. However I discovered that sharing my feelings and thoughts was very beneficial for me.

175

WHAT YOU CAN DO TO MAKE IT EASIER FOR YOU AND YOUR SUPPORT SYSTEM

Tell them how you're feeling.
- The only way people can understand what you're thinking or feeling is if you tell them.

Don't lie about your pain.
- Close family and friends may not ask how you're doing every time they see you. On the days that they don't ask and you want or need to talk about it, let them know.

Ask for help when you need it.
- As it was with me, you probably were taught to value your independence, so it may be difficult for you to ask for help. But sometimes we all need help. Try asking in a way that explains what's going on.

Be a cheerful receiver.
- When someone helps you or gives you a sincere compliment about your progress, say "Thanks." It is OK to need help or an emotional boost.

Allow Family and friends to help.
- Most likely, your family and friends have asked you what they can do to help you. Maybe you didn't know what to say or you felt negatively about letting others know you needed any type of special treatment. It is possible that your family and friends have decided to help in ways that irritate you. Perhaps they assume they're making you feel better, but if they're not it is important that you let them know.

SIX THINGS YOU COULD SAY WHEN PEOPLE ASK YOU IF THERE IS ANYTHING THEY CAN DO FOR YOU.

1. "Learn about cancer"
- Learning about cancer will give family and friends insight .

into what you're going through, how they can help and when they shouldn't help. For example when friends and family members take charge of something that you can do on your own, they unintentionally wear away your independence and self-confidence.

2. "Please don't let all our conversations be about me"
   • It's easy for friends and family to get caught up in discussing your cancer. But that only reminds you of your condition, and that is something you don't want to do.

3. "Try not to be too overly attentive to me"
   • Being overly helpful to someone with an illness actually can slow down healing. Let people know that you appreciate their concern, but you don't need a servant. To manage, you need to learn to do things for yourself again. Many studies confirm that when family members are supportive without reinforcing the illness, the person has a much better prognosis.

4. "Come with me to appointments; go for walks with me"
   • When friends and family members go with you on walks and to doctor visits or support group meetings, it can be very helpful for both of you. It gives you and the other person a chance to talk and share time together. It also gives the other person an opportunity to learn more about the importance for you to exercise and stay active.

5. "Please to listen to me"
   • Sometimes all you need is for someone to listen. A family member or friend can give you emotional support that allows you to release your stresses. People who feel they have support of family and friends cope better with their pain, live more active lives, and return to work earlier. Your family members and friends can help you by reminding you of the progress you're making and keeping you focused on positive solutions to your problems.

6. "Please take care of yourself"
   • Your condition affects your friends and family members. They, worry, feel depression, and suffer from exhaustion. Remind those you care about to take care of their own health, as well.

DRAGON BOAT TEAMS FOR WOMEN WITH BREAST CANCER

A few months before I was diagnosed with breast cancer, in the same year the first breast cancer survivor dragon boat team was launched in Vancouver, Canada in February 1996. Dr. Don McKenzie, a sports medicine physician at the University of British Columbia, launched *Abreast In A Boat* in 1996 to test the myth that repetitive upper-body exercise in women treated for breast cancer encourages lymphedema.

Dr McKenzie believed that by following a special exercise and training program, women could avoid lymphedema and enjoy active, full lives. Dr McKenzie's theory was proven correct. No new cases of lymphedema occurred and none of the existing cases became worse. This was also true for me. When I joined the dragon boat team, I had already developed lymphedema and the exercise I received from dragon boating did not make my lymphedema worse.

Women recovering from and battling breast cancer are now paddling Dragon Boats all over the world. For years, doctors warned breast cancer patients to avoid strenuous upper body workouts. Canadian researchers have found that paddling is not only safe, it is actually good for breast cancer patients. Women who have been treated for breast cancer are at a greater risk of cardiovascular disease and osteoporosis, so an upper body workout is important to keep us healthy.

I discovered there are no consistent strategies for survivors of breast cancer. Recommendations about physical activity were mostly information about what I should not to do instead of what I could do. Physical activity affects the production, metabolism, and release of female hormones. It also affects our energy, and this may be linked to the lower risk of breast cancer in women who exercise regularly.

Dragon boating for people with breast cancer was chosen for many reasons. It is a strenuous, repetitive upper body activity that sends a visible message to all people with breast cancer.

In many ways, it is an ideal exercise. It is non-weight-bearing and, therefore, is associated with a lower risk of injury than weight-dependent activities, such as running. It is safe, and with proper technique, the paddler can build a fair amount of muscle mass and make positive changes in the musculoskeletal and cardiovascular systems.

It uses mostly upper body and trunk muscles, and the improvement in strength has a carry-over effect to day-to-day activity. The training intensity can be changed simply by pulling harder. This is important because, with a wide range in ages and athletic abilities, each paddler can still have a training effect.

Dragon boating is a team sport that builds harmony and a feeling of togetherness. It looks good, and is honest physical work that results in obvious improvements in fitness.

A dragon boat can hold 22–26 paddlers, and this gives women a chance to work with a large group at one time. Above all, dragon boating is exciting!

HOW TO JOIN A BREAST CANCER DRAGON BOAT TEAM

Usually the only criterion for joining a breast cancer dragon boat team is that you have a history of breast cancer. How old you are and how athletic your are and whether or not you have ever participated in dragon boating does not matter. The 24 paddlers in the boat I was in ranged in age from 21 to 75 years.

ANTIOXIDANTS

An antioxidant is a chemical that prevents the oxidation of other chemicals. In biological systems, the normal processes of oxidation (plus a minor contribution from ionizing radiation) produce highly reactive free radicals. These can readily react with and damage other molecules: In some cases, the body uses this to fight infection; in other cases, the damage may continue to the body's own cells. The presence of readily oxidisable compounds(antioxidants) in the system can "mop up" free radicals before they damage other essential molecules. Many forms of cancer are thought to be the result of reactions between free radicals and DNA, resulting in mutations that can adversely affect the cell cycle and potentially lead to malignancy.

WHAT IS CANCER?

Cancer is defined as a disease that causes cells in the body to change and multiply out of control, disrupting the normal function of a particular organ or organs. Cancer begins when the DNA molecules—the materials in our cells that dictate our genetic makeup and control the way our cells divide—are altered. Cancer cells then begin to grow and multiply, often forming tumors that may damage or destroy normal tissue. Not all tumors are cancerous: Benign tumors do not grow and spread like cancer, and they usually don't become a serious health threat.

Cancer is a disease process in which healthy cells stop functioning and maturing properly. As the normal cycle of cell creation and death is interrupted, the newly mutated cancer cells begin multiplying uncontrollably, no longer operating as an integrated and harmonious part of the body. In its simplest terms, cancer represents an accelerating process of inappropriate, uncontrolled cell growth—a chaotic process within the order of biology. Normally, DNA mutations are repaired or made harmless by the immune system.

Every one of us, every day, creates hundreds of thousands of cancer cells usually recognized and destroyed by our immune systems.

When genetic mutations remain uncorrected—and this will happen when the immune system is not effective due to its being suppressed, weakened, or overwhelmed—then a cancer process can potentially move to its next stage of uncontrolled rapid growth. It does this by making copies of itself, a normal function of DNA; except in this case, the mutated and undesirable DNA is copying itself. As more cancer cells grow, the process continues to multiply to form a tumor.

The normal order of cell growth, duplication and separation then become disorderly, leading to chaos in the body.

INNER VOICE, INNER KNOWING

What does it mean? Where does it come from? For those who know it and who have listened to it themselves, they will understand what I am talking about. But others, for whom this concept is new, will question what it is and how to know which inner "voice" to listen to. I've heard it explained, and I agree with what I heard, that a part of us is connected to our higher self. Our higher self is connected to not only the universe, but also to the higher power we call God, Spirit, The Force, Creator, and many other names. I know that when I connect to that part of myself, the information which seems to flow through me is not emotional; it may not seem rational, either, but there are no emotions attached to it. With it comes a deep sense of calm and a deep sense of knowingness and peace. I know what it is not. It is not the voice of your conscience; it is not your parents' voices still giving you direction—it is bigger and higher and deeper and larger. It is ageless and timeless and interconnected; I believe that it has access to everything and anything.

THE SUPPLEMENTS I TOOK AND THE DIET CHANGES I MADE:

• I took massive doses of Vitamin C (10,000 mg @ day) to boost my immune system. Vitamin C helps our body's natural defense against cancer. Vitamin C works by preventing tumor growth and helping resist formation of metastases (the spreading of cancer cells to other parts of the body). It further improves our immune system's functioning by playing a role in the production of interferons and aiding white blood cells in their work. Antioxidants help destroy the free radical cells, and antioxidants, in small amounts, will inhibit the combining of oxygen with other compounds.

• I drank Essiac tea to purify my blood. Essiac is a mixture of four herbs. Indian rhubarb, sheep head sorrel, slippery elm, and burdock root. Essiac tea strengthens the body's immune system, allowing it to fight cancer. It improves appetite, supplies vitamins, enzymes, and minerals, relieves pain, and may prolong life. One of the herbs in Essiac tea decreases tumor growth and the others act as blood purifiers. Essiac Tea is beneficial for many types of cancer, including breast cancer.

• Shark cartilage helps capsulate the tumor and prevent it from growing. Here is how it works. As a tumor grows, it develops a network of blood vessels that provide it with the necessary blood supply and energy to survive and grow. This process is called angiogenesis. Shark cartilage prevents blood vessels from forming. As a result, the tumor starves because it does not get the blood and nutrients it needs. Shark cartilage works best on solid tumors, as they need a lot of new blood vessels to grow. This includes breast cancer, as well as tumors of the central nervous system, cervix, prostate and pancreas.

• I took Coenzyme Q10, which suppresses the proliferation of cancer cells. Research indicates that Coenzyme Q10 also boosts the Immune System chemicals that attack cancer cells.

• I changed my diet drastically to avoid dairy products, artificial and refined sugar, refined or processed products, caffeine, alcohol, beef, pork, deep fried foods (heated oils); and food containing additives, preservatives, or food coloring. My diet was an alkaline/acid cleansing diet. This type of diet is important for us to have a balanced body chemistry in order to maintain good health and eliminate disease. Too much acid in our body tissue is one of the basic causes of cancer cell growth and spread. It is important that there is a proper ratio between acid and alkaline foods in our diet. For example, fruits, vegetables and a few legumes form an alkaline ash in our body, while all other foods form an acid ash. The natural ratio in a normal healthy body is approximately four to one—four parts alkaline to one part acid. When an ideal ratio is maintained, our body has a strong resistance to cancer. In healing, the higher the ratio of alkaline in the diet, the faster the recovery. Food is to be organic, whenever possible, and fruit and vegetables make up the bulk of the diet.

• I drank green tea. Green tea neutralizes free radicals, which are believed to lead to cancer.

• I took blue green algae. Spirulina is unicellular blue - green algae that has been consumed by humans since ancient times in Mexico and Africa. It is currently grown in many countries by synthetic methods. Initially, Spirulina was eaten for its nutritive value. It is a rich natural source of proteins, carotenoids, and other micronutrients. Recent preclinical testing suggests it may have immunological, antiviral, and cholesterol-reducing therapeutic properties. In animal experiments for short-term and long-term toxicity, mutagenicity, and teratogenicity, the algae did not cause toxicity. The Spirulina administered to the animals in the studies were at much higher amounts than those expected in human consumption. Research in Japan has shown that the substance phycocyanin in spirulina raises lymphocyte activity and strengthens the immune system. In India and Germany, researchers have used spirulina to reduce cholesterol levels and to lower blood pressure in those with mild hypertension.

• I took Echinacea. Echinacea is a flower that belongs to the sunflower family. Supporters claim that Echinacea increases the number and activity of cells in our immune system. As a result, our immune system is thought to be stimulated and better able to fight disease. It is not known, exactly, which compounds in Echinacea might be responsible for such immune enhancement.

HISTORY OF THE DRAGON BOAT

Dragon Boat racing is part of the Chinese Culture. Every year on the fifth day of the fifth moon of the lunar calendar, people celebrate the Duan Yang (High Noon) Festival. It is a fertility festival in which people ask for rain and a good harvest. During the festival, Dragon Boat races are organized.

The High Noon Festival is the most important festival after the New Year. In the Hunan province of China, Dragon Boats are kept in nearby temples. A couple of days before the festival, the boats are ceremonially pulled out of their storage and a Dragon Head and Tail are mounted. Offerings are made to the spirits before the boats are put into the water. The dragon is ritually awakened. A Taotic priest blesses the boat and colors the eyes of the Dragon Head as the Dragon awakens.

The Dragon Boat race derives from the death of Qu Yuan, a poet-philosopher who committed suicide by jumping into the Mei Lo River to protest the corrupt regime of a Chou emperor. According to legend, local fishermen, upon seeing their beloved poet's act of courage, raced out in their boats in an attempt to save his life. They arrived too late, but to prevent the fish from eating his body they beat the water furiously with their paddles and threw rice dumplings wrapped in silk into the river to distract the fish. A re-enactment of this legend is conducted at Dragon Boat racing events.

BOOKS THAT WERE IMPORTANT TO ME

Love, Medicine and Miracle, by Bernie S. Siegel, M. D.

Peace, Love & Healing, by Bernie S. Siegel, M. D.

Dr. Susan Love's Breast Book, by: Susan M. Love, M. D. with Karen Lindsey

Alternative Medicine the Definitive Guide, compiled by The Burton Goldberg Group, Future Medicine Publishing Inc.

New Choices in Natural Healing, Rodale Press Inc.

Psychosynthesis, by Roberto Assagioli, M. D.

Anatomy of an illness, by Norman Cousins

Ageless Body, Timeless Mind, by Deepak Chopra, M. D.

SOME THOUGHTS ON MAINSTREAM MEDICINE VS ALTERNATIVE MEDICINE

Medical practice was not always so tightly connected to science. As little as two centuries ago medicine was more based on a belief system of what worked based on evidence; research was infrequent and uncoordinated and it was not generally accepted as the way to improve the practice of medicine.

Slowly, however, a few scientists began to use research and experimentation and this showed how factual knowledge could be used to treat and cure patients. Medical research increased and one by one, diseases began to fall under the understanding and control of mainstream medical doctors, and the results are undeniable.

Today, medical research is a multi-billion dollar industry.

Many alternative treatments are based on anecdotal experiences. Mainstream doctors view anecdotal experience as weak. Why? In part, it is because human biology is extremely complex and variable. The fact is that no two patients are exactly alike and, therefore, the results are never completely predictable.

For anecdotal records doctors rely heavily on the patient's personal experience of their own disease and symptoms.

Doctors think that they can only know how much pain patients experience by what they tell them; there is no objective measure. Patient's expectations, the so-called placebo effect, are very powerful and greatly affect a person's beliefs about whether or not they are getting better or worse. A doctor's belief is also a factor, if they believe a patient should be getting better, their assessment of them may be influenced in that direction.

The FDA was established to protect the public from so-called snake oil salesman, slick con-artists who sold useless or even harmful concoctions with a long list of unsubstantiated health claims.

Doctors of mainstream medicine often consider themselves *healers*. I believe this view is incorrect. Doctors cannot heal their patients: Only patients can heal themselves. Doctors can, at most, assist or complicate healing.

Alternative medicine puts a great deal of trust in the functioning of the human life form. If a person gets what our human body expects and needs, he/she will be healthy and thrive. Alternative medicine believes that Dis-Ease is a symptom of a system out of balance. Re-balance the system and the symptom will likely disappear.

Alternative medicine tries to discover and correct dietary deficiencies, unhealthy habits, emotional stresses, and environmental toxins that bring disorder in the human system. Alternative medicine tries to nurture and stimulate the body's immune system to help it do its job, and it deals with serious symptoms in a way that has little or no negative effect on the rest of the human system.

The idea of *balance* is common in philosophies of Alternative medicine (as opposed to science based Mainstream medicine). The treatments I feel strongest about all have their philosophies of health and wellness based on balance. This is especially true for Chiropractic care and Psychosynthesis.

ACKNOWLEDGMENTS

To Paul, for all your continuous love and support, without you, life would have less meaning and I would be less whole.

To Vincent, you are the greatest gift of all. Being your mother gives my life a richness and depth that continues to amaze me.

To Liesbeth, Anneke, Michelle, Jacqueline, Alice, Jenni and Linda for taking time to read the pages and giving me your thoughts. Your support and excitement is very important to me.

To Jerre Paquette and Carole Jeffries, for doing an astonishing editing job. Your comments made the book much better, especially the ones about the commas. Thanks you two!

To Ieke, Jenni and Dan, for your friendship and for showing me the importance of having a support team and a cheering section.

To Julie for your guidance, insight, friendship and unselfish support.

A heartfelt thanks to all of you who shared this part of my journey, naming you individually would fill another book. Your support nurtured and empowered me.

To my family doctor for being a team player instead of a puppet master.

To my siblings: Marian, Liesbeth, Anneke, Joan and Neil for showing me the importance of family.

And a very special thanks to Stephen Jones, for all your unconditional support!

ISBN 141207993-4